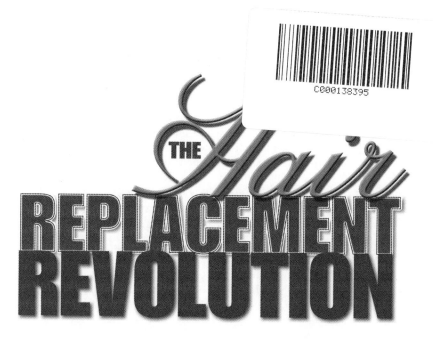

THE *Hair* REPLACEMENT REVOLUTION

A Consumer's Guide to Effective Hair Replacement Techniques

JAMES HARRIS, MD
EMANUEL MARRITT, MD

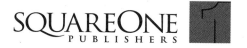

SQUAREONE
PUBLISHERS

The information and advice in this book are based on the training, personal experiences, and research of the authors. Its contents are current and accurate; however, the information presented is not intended to substitute for professional medical advice. The authors and the publisher urge you to consult with your physician or other qualified health-care provider prior to starting any treatment or undergoing any surgical procedure. Because there is always some risk involved, the authors and publisher cannot be responsible for any adverse effects or consequences resulting from the use of any of the suggestions, preparations, or procedures described in this book.

COVER DESIGNER: Phaedra Mastrocola • COVER PHOTO: SuperStock, Inc.
IN-HOUSE EDITOR: Marie Caratozzolo • TYPESETTER: Gary A. Rosenberg

Square One Publishers
115 Herricks Road
Garden City Park, NY 11040
(516) 535-2010 • (877) 900-BOOK
www.squareonepublishers.com

Library of Congress Cataloging-in-Publication Data

Harris, James, M.D.
    The hair replacement revolution : a consumer's guide to effective hair replacement techniques / James Harris, Emanuel Marritt.
        p. ; cm.
    Includes bibliographical references and index.
    ISBN 0-7570-0004-5 (pbk.)
    1. Baldness—Treatment.
        [DNLM: 1. Hair—transplantation—Popular Works. 2. Alopecia—Popular Works. 3. Reconstructive Surgical Procedures—methods—Popular Works. WR 450 H314h 2003] I. Marritt, Emanuel. II. Title.
    RL155.H37   2003
    616.5'46—dc21

                                                                    2002156167

Contents

Part III The Right Decision

Acknowledgments

It is with great appreciation that we recognize those individuals who helped in the production of this book. We must thank our families and friends, who kept asking, "Are you finished yet?" You provided encouragement and support. We must also thank physicians Dr. Michael Beehner, Dr. Robert Bernstein, Dr. Sharon Keene, Dr. Keith Kaufman, Dr. Bobby Limmer, Dr. Bradley Limmer, Dr. Bernard Nusbaum, Dr. Elise Olsen, Dr. William Parsley, Dr. William Reed, Dr. William Rassman, and Dr. Walter Unger for their contributions, which came in many forms—pearls of information, helpful criticisms, photograph usage, and simple support. We must thank Mr. Peter Friedaur of Züri SalonSpa of Denver, Colorado, for lending his input on styling considerations. We are also very grateful to Mr. Mike Mahoney of www.IWantHair.com for his professional assistance in simplifying the complexities of hair additions. Special thanks to Mr. Tony Lauro for his assistance in preparing the manuscript and for helping with the background research. Thanks to our publisher, Mr. Rudy Shur, for his expertise, as well as his recognition of the importance of a book of this type. We would like to express gratitude to our editor, Ms. Marie Caratozzolo, for her unwavering enthusiasm, patience, editorial acumen, and perseverance. A special thanks goes to the office staff, especially Shanee Courtney, RN, BSN, for the countless number of times they assisted us throughout this project; we are very lucky to have had your help.

Foreword

I n the thirty-six years I have been transplanting hair, I have taught hundreds of physicians from all over the world, Dr. Emanuel Marritt amongst them. His combination of intelligence, enthusiasm, attention to detail, openness to new ideas, and high ethics were obvious and unique in my experience. This book "for non-physicians" by Dr. Marritt and Dr. James Harris, the man he chose from amongst many to take over his clinical practice, is not only an outstanding gift to the public, it is a gift to all hair replacement specialists.

The Hair Replacement Revolution is a work that is long overdue. It offers the very important first step for anyone who is interested in a treatment option for hair loss. From my many years in this field, I know only too well the problems that can occur when an individual has not done sufficient research before choosing a hair loss treatment. I have seen first-hand the devastating and permanent disfigurements that can result from improper surgical treatments. I also know scores of people who have spent their time and money on cosmetic hair additions, only to be disappointed by systems that were either poorly constructed or inappropriately designed for their age or facial structure. No less upsetting to me is having to continually witness the growing parade of hopeful individuals who are willing to ingest any pill or elixir, try any topical cream or shampoo, or use any product that promises to give them the hair that they desire.

Through their collaborative effort, Drs. Harris and Marritt have provided a book that objectively guides the reader through the physical realities of hair loss, provides the truth about the legitimate available treatment alternatives (the positives as well as the negatives), and increases consumer awareness of industry falsehoods. Their work offers a wealth of information for anyone who wants answers to pertinent hair restoration questions in order to avoid potential traumas or disappointments.

A unique blend of science and artistry, the field of hair replacement surgery has grown exponentially over the past few decades. As co-editor of the 2003 edition of *Hair Transplantation*, I can attest to the fact that it is a constantly evolving procedure in a field whose scientific and technological advancements are ever-changing. Although my views on some of the information presented may differ somewhat from those of Drs. Harris and Marritt, this book is the perfect starting place for those who seek a clear and honest presentation of the facts. In a further effort to help readers research their options, keep up with current news, and locate professionals in the field, Drs. Harris and Marritt have also included a list of resources, including helpful websites. Keep in mind, however, that there are dozens of qualified professionals who may not be listed on these sites. By reading this book and learning how to ask the right questions, readers will be able to find both the right process and best hair restoration professional to meet their needs.

A hair replacement revolution can be as good *or bad* as any "revolution." Your best friend is this book.

Walter Unger, MD
Co-editor of *Hair Restoration*, 2003 edition
New York, NY

Introduction

The attractive guy on the cover of this book delivers an unspoken promise of youth, good looks, and lots of hair! It is an irresistible image that is typical of those used in ads and brochures and commercials in the hair-loss industry—one that has been created to finesse consumers into plunking down their hard-earned money and buying into a dream. Unfortunately, the hair loss industry is and has always been a target for snake-oil salesmen and slick marketers who prey on the vulnerability of people who are desperate for a "cure." The marketplace is filled with lotions and potions and "breakthrough advances" that promise to deliver the hair that is so desirable and in such demand. And consumers are instantly drawn to that possibility, unable to resist the possible realization of their hopes. Sadly, however, after throwing away precious dollars chasing that elusive dream, they come to the eventual reality that the promise didn't live up to its claim. Disheartened, they may come away from the experience a little wiser, but quickly abandon that wisdom when the next "miracle cure" comes along.

Of course, not all hair loss treatments and alternatives fall into the "suspicious" category. There have been a number of extraordinary advances in this field. If you are one of the millions looking to separate the fact from the fiction, the truth from the exaggeration, you have come to the right place. This book is all about the truth. It is designed to cut through the misleading ads and promotions that continually bombard the marketplace, and focus on the realities of hair restoration.

1

When dealing with any major decision, the more information you have, the better able you will be to make the right choice. Seems pretty straightforward, doesn't it? Well, it is and it isn't. Every book, every magazine article contains information. Every advertisement, brochure, video, or infomercial contains *some* kind of information. But when it comes to treating hair loss, the most critical task is determining the *legitimacy* of that information. With collective careers of over thirty-five years as hair-replacement surgeons, we were determined through this book to deliver the accurate, honest information that you, the consumer, should expect and deserve. Our goal was to enlighten and educate.

So what's in this book? *The Hair Replacement Revolution* is a user-friendly practical guide that clearly and objectively presents information on all aspects of hair loss, from its physical causes and psychological ramifications, to its many legitimate and not-so-legitimate treatment options. It takes you by the hand, and helps you focus on the best personal choices for your particular situation. Divided into three main parts, the book begins with a section on hair-loss basics, moves on to the various options in dealing with hair loss, and then closes with guidelines on how to make the best decision for your particular situation.

The first chapter in Part I offers a brief history of the evolution of the hair-replacement field, from its early roots to its incredible explosion into the ever-growing multibillion-dollar industry it is today. As you will see, the technological advances in all three branches—surgical, cosmetic, and pharmaceutical—are nothing less than astounding. Along with this success, however, also lurks industry fraud and misrepresentation. In this opening chapter and throughout the book, your eyes will be opened to many of the scams, unethical practices, and even the dangers found within the field. In an effort to help you better understand yourself and your personal reaction to hair loss, Chapter 2 discusses common psychological factors (often subtle, yet powerful) that are associated with this condition. You'll learn how to handle the fear, confusion, and anxiety that characteristically plagues those who are dealing with baldness. You'll discover how the right attitude is crucial in achieving the best outcome in your search for hair. Chapter 3 concludes this section by outlining the various types of hair loss. It begins with some basic information on the anatomy and life cycle of the hair follicle, and then goes on to dispel the common myths that are believed to trigger hair loss, while clearly explaining its true causes.

Part II is all about hair-replacement options. The chapters in this section offer comprehensive information on the legitimate choices that are available for dealing with hair loss, including the decision to do nothing at all. That's right. Staying bald is a viable choice that you just may determine is best for you. Chapter 4 welcomes you to the world of cosmetic hair additions. By the time you have reached the end of this chapter, you'll know everything about them—their basic components, the different attachment methods, and why some appear more natural than others. Pharmaceuticals that have been scientifically tested and approved for the treatment of hair loss are presented in Chapter 5, along with a warning about the unending parade of products that "claim" hair-growth success. Chapter 6 is an all-inclusive chapter on surgical options that details the pros and cons of various hair-restoring procedures, focusing special attention on the latest transplantation techniques. A discussion on bogus surgical procedures that you should be aware of and avoid concludes the chapter. And for those who are in need of repair or reconstruction—often the result of poorly performed prior surgeries—Chapter 7 presents the procedures used to remedy these problems.

While the first two sections of *The Hair Replacement Revolution* provide all of the necessary information on hair loss and its available options, Part III is designed to aid you in your decision-making. Are you going to accept your hair loss, or will you attempt to replace it? And if your decision is the latter, which option seems best for you? A hair addition? A surgical procedure? A pharmaceutical therapy? Chapter 8 examines a variety of factors regarding these options that must be considered, such as the time and cost involved, as well as your personal preferences. This evaluation will help you focus on your particular needs in making the right choice. By the time you reach Chapter 9, there's a good chance that you may want to investigate further one or more of the hair-restoration options. This last chapter will aid you in the search for a qualified provider who can help you achieve your goal. Not only does it offer suggestions for locating hair-replacement professionals, it also outlines essential guidelines for helping in your assessment of them. Rounding out this chapter is some solid advice that will help you see through all of the hype that's out there—the special offers, the claims that seem too good to be true, the amazing but suspicious before-and-after photos, and more.

The Hair Replacement Revolution offers knowledge, and knowledge is power. It will arm you with all of the information, support, and skill you'll need to become a savvy consumer—someone who is prepared to objectively and realistically assess all of the possible alternatives. Most important, it will empower you with the confidence to make the right decision. If you have gained this strength and confidence after reading this book, we will have done our job.

PART I

The Background

1

The Business of Hair Loss

"You can fool all of the people all of the time . . .
if the advertising budget is big enough."

—ED ROLLINS, POLITICAL ADVISOR

The times have certainly changed for the field of hair replacement. Over the years, as cosmetic surgery has gained acceptance, the popularity of hair replacement has risen as well. It is a golden age for the entire field. In an industry that now grosses more than a billion dollars annually, the technological advances in all three branches—surgical, cosmetic, and pharmaceutical—are nothing less than astounding.

Although we are in the middle of the hair replacement's technological and financial golden age, it is also the age of big business, multinational chains, and direct-market advertising. Along with this comes hair-transplant "counselors," video sales pitches, and unwanted phone solicitation. To avoid industry fraud, misrepresentation, and, worst of all, disfigurement, anyone interested in hair replacement must become educated.

Never have more choices been available, and yet, never have more outrageous promises been made, directly impeding the consumer's ability to choose among the many options. This chapter, therefore, is about realigning your attitude towards the field of hair replacement. It will help raise your awareness level of the misrepresentations and even dangers found within the industry. In other words, it will help you become a savvy consumer.

O'Tar Norwood, MD, a prominent hair-replacement surgeon from Oklahoma City and author of several textbooks, has cautioned that "[we] must be careful, ethical, and truthful. It is very easy to emphasize the positive things about a procedure and ignore, or de-emphasize the negative aspects. We must be very careful because it is very easy when dealing with hair and aesthetics to mislead an under-educated consumer." This is an excellent reminder that applies to all three areas of the hair-replacement field. To ensure that you are not misled, this chapter will reveal some of the unsavory business practices that have permeated this field. Don't worry, though, many ethical doctors and other hair-replacement professionals still exist. But an important first step in helping to identify the best in the field is learning to avoid those people, products, and practices that will *not* help you reach your goals.

BAD BUSINESS PRACTICES

Business has always been a part of medicine. Even Hippocrates, the father of modern medicine who lived in ancient Greece, had to charge for procedures and sell tonics to cover his expenses. In the 1800s, traveling salesmen sold snake oils and tonics to anyone willing to hand over a few pennies, and even in the 1950s—a perceived golden age in America—there were unethical doctors and salesmen who conned people out of their money. What is most important to remember about those times is that the vast majority of doctors, salesmen, and others who dispensed medical information and services were relatively ethical. But some time in the early 1980s, the balance in the field of hair replacement changed, and the number of people trying to take advantage of hair clients grew, eventually appearing to constitute the majority in the field.

As this balance shifted, the profession of surgical hair replacement was transformed into a business, with the search for profits—not a search for healing—as the driving force. Unfortunately, the patient or client was transformed into a consumer. The difference between profession and business, patient and consumer is enormous. A patient seeks out a doctor for trustworthy advice on how to cure an ailment, and the doctor gives his opinion based on years of experience and training. The patient assumes that the physician places his well-being above all other considerations. A consumer, on the other hand, goes to a place of business and talks with a salesperson. The salesperson gives his biased opinion, hoping to sell another "widget," whether or not the consumer needs it or wants it. The consumer understands the sales process and, therefore, approaches the relationship with caution. The biggest problem with the change from profession to business is that most people who have experienced hair loss don't even realize the change has taken place.

SURGICAL HAIR REPLACEMENT

The surgical branch of the hair-replacement field is the area in which the invasion of business tactics has had the most impact. This is largely because the consequences are so much greater. Losing money is certainly serious, but not more so than permanent scarring and disfigurement. Since the 1980s, over 50 percent of our patients have come to us in need of repair and reconstruction because of poor results from inferior transplant surgery. Many of these patients just wanted to look normal enough to be seen in public. This was truly sad, because their disfigurements could have been prevented.

Why are so many hair-replacement patients failing to get the results they want and expect? As you are about to see, there are a number of contributing factors.

Doctors Find You

In the 1970s, when the surgical hair-replacement field was still in its infancy, prospective patients usually asked their family general practitioner, a dermatologist, or even the local medical school for referrals of competent hair-replacement surgeons—in effect, an endorsement by a trusted source. Furthermore, because the referring parties had no vested financial interest in the outcome, they could give accurate, unbiased information to the best of their knowledge and expertise. With this initial recommendation, the patient then scheduled a consultation with the surgeon.

Today, without rules prohibiting medical advertising, to find a hair-replacement surgeon, one can simply log onto the Internet, scan the sports pages of the newspaper, or watch infomercials.

Each of these avenues usually leads to the same place—an 800 number, from which the caller will receive a brochure and an "informational" video. These methods circumvent the traditional safeguards for finding a surgeon.

But the lack of safeguards doesn't end there. Most people then go to consultations still expecting ethical, factual, and objective advice regarding the treatment of hair loss. However, many consultation offices have changed from straightforward sources of information into seductive showrooms—so cleverly designed and disguised that, to the trusting patient, they appear to be doctors' offices. Ingrid Wagner-Smith, MBA, CMR, a hair-replacement technician from St. Louis, laments, "Unfortunately . . . the patient can no longer distinguish gimmick and hype from fact."

Advertising, however, is now something of a necessary evil, because it is difficult for novice surgeons to get patients without advertising in some way. Traditionally, a doctor, at least in part, built up a practice through personal referrals. Satisfied patients were—and still are—a surgeon's best and least expensive form of advertising. Unfortunately, these traditional methods take time to have any effect. Unlike other forms of cosmetic surgery, hair transplantation can require one or two years for completion. So what does the novice hair-replacement surgeon do to establish a practice while waiting for his first patients' hair to grow out? He advertises.

Of course, advertising can be responsible, ethical, and educational. It can create increased consumer awareness and healthy competition, which, in turn, can act as a force to improve technology, decrease fees, and increase the availability of state-of-the-art procedures. Unfortunately, some doctors and clinics take a different approach; they will use any gimmick or unrealistic promise to get new patients.

Promises That a Scalpel Can't Keep

Russell Knudsen, MD, past President of both the International Society of Hair Replacement Surgery and the Australian Society of Hair Replacement Surgeons in Sydney, Australia, once warned, "Never let your mouth make promises that your scalpel can't keep." The fact is, however, that unethical hair-replacement surgeons do make promises that can't be kept. They promise clients the complete return of *all* lost hair—as much hair as they want, as fast as they want it. Unfortunately, hair-replacement surgeons do not and cannot replace, restore, revive, or resuscitate dead and departed hair. They can only take permanently growing hair from the back and sides of a head and redistribute it over the bald areas on the top and front. No patient has one more hair on his head in his "after" picture than he did in his "before" picture. It just looks as if he does. His hair has been rearranged, not replaced.

While this fact may limit your expectations of the hair-replacement process, it does not mean that you can't get great results. It just means that, contrary to what some doctors may promise, you can't have it all.

The Rise of Multi-Center Clinics

Multi-center or chain clinics specializing in hair-replacement surgery have taken the place of many traditional doctors' offices. It is difficult to say exactly what provides the impetus for such a trend, but it would be safe to assume that "profit" is a major force. Although these multi-center establishments can provide excellent results, they are not without certain inherent problems, which are presented in the following discussions.

Who Works in Multi-Center Clinics?

Many people assume that multi-center clinics are on the cutting edge of technology. Whether or not this is true, the clinic itself is not the issue. The two essential elements of surgery are always you and your surgeon. It is an individual doctor, not a clinic or institute, who operates on your head. So it is the surgeon who must have the competence to perform the procedure that you have chosen.

Of course, the clinic will try to convince you that its surgeons are all masters of their craft. But consider this: If a clinic is overflowing with such gifted, artistic, leading authorities, why are they working there? Typically, less experienced doctors work at these clinics, trying to gain experience without the stress of managing a private practice. And nothing is inherently wrong or even unethical about doctors working for other doctors. In some instances, a surgeon can spend more time conducting research or writing professional articles if someone else runs the business. However, this scenario is the exception rather than the rule.

Moreover, nothing is wrong with your choosing to go to a clinic for many reasons, including cost, convenience, and location. Some people do receive good, satisfying results from multi-center clinic surgeons. What's critical, however, is to evaluate the clinic and its surgeons before making any commitments. The information found in this book will help guide you in this evaluation.

Who Pays the Overhead?

Inherent within any doctor's practice are the ongoing responsibilities of managing personnel, patient records, office overhead, and bookkeeping. Any doctor who decides to expand his practice into a national chain will be responsible for vastly increased overhead. He will sign multiple leases and hire and train many new employees, including other doctors. Most important, he will significantly increase his advertising budget. Because these expenses are paid up front, they can become either a subtle or a not so subtle pressure to increase income.

In the largest nationally franchised institutes, the advertising budgets can be counted in the millions of dollars for a single year, sometimes exceeding $10 million according to the trade journal *Ad Week*. Remember, that's $10 million in addition to the standard expenses, including doctors' fees, nurses' salaries, rent, supplies, and medications. So, by the time you walk through the door of the clinic, you are not viewed only as a patient, but also as an expense to be covered. The income to cover such monumental expenses comes from one place only—surgery performed on your head.

Doctors will acknowledge this potential conflict of interest, but many will counter with, "I can handle it." Yet it is not easy to do so. Only one reason compels doctors to advertise—to increase their number of patients. The patient-consumer needs to be aware that there may be a direct correlation between the amount of advertising that a clinic does and the pressure that it may place on the patient to have surgery performed. The feeling that one is being pressured, coerced, or "sold" should be a warning sign that perhaps your best interest is not the top priority of the physician or clinic.

"Counselors" Replace Doctors

The expansion of the traditional doctor's office into a multi-center clinic has given rise to another new development—the hair-replacement counselor. As the surgeon feels the pressure to earn more money to pay for increasing overhead, he must spend more of his time operating, thereby generating more income. From an economic perspective, his most valuable time is surgical time. As a result, others may be responsible for some of the tasks that have been traditionally performed by doctors, including the most time-consuming but also most important task: the consultation.

To solve the surgeon's operating room-versus-consultation room dilemma, many clinics now use hair-replacement counselors. These "counselors" are often nothing more than salesmen in white lab coats, working on commission. Posing as qualified medical advisers, these "professionals" represent the doctor in consultations. They may even plan the new hairline, diagnose the future extent of baldness, and assess donor graft availability. Prospective patients should be aware that these counselors are not licensed in any field of medical practice to give out surgical recommendations of any kind. Only a surgeon is qualified to make such suggestions.

Ideally, the doctor and his patient, after proper discussion in search of a common but realistic goal, should form a strong and lasting bond. Unfortunately, such bonds are strikingly absent from many doctor-patient relationships, which have been reduced to consent forms and payment plans. The bond between a surgeon and patient cannot even begin to form when a counselor-salesman substitutes for the doctor during the consultation.

Substituting a counselor for a doctor is distressing enough, but it is only the first step toward an eroding doctor-patient relationship. In many cases, the patient first meets the doctor on the day of surgery, and often during the presurgical preparation. There's a good chance that any patient who meets the surgeon on the day of the operation has not been made sufficiently aware of all treatment options, has not had the opportunity to understand the nature of his condition, and doesn't have the proper expectations for the outcome of the surgery.

Assessing the skill and compassion of a surgeon is hard enough under the best of circumstances—and it's nearly impossible to do immediately prior to surgery. Although in the final analysis, it doesn't matter whether a surgeon is deliberate in his deceptions, or just plain naive and unaware of the ramifications of surgical hair replacement, the end result can be the same. Therefore, knowing your surgeon and his attitude towards surgery is vital in order to achieve a safe and satisfying result. It is a process that takes time.

Understanding the element of time is as important as understanding the surgery itself. Meeting your surgeon in the operating room for the first time is perfectly appropriate if you've just been in a car accident and suffered some serious trauma that needs immediate attention. Certainly, this would hardly be the time to ask for your surgeon's credentials or to request a meeting with some of his other patients. Elective or cosmetic surgery, conversely, is, by definition, a choice. There should be no feeling of urgency.

Clinics Become Superstores

A number of hair-replacement clinics have become superstores. They offer all of the options—surgical, pharmaceutical, and cosmetic. These places claim that because they offer everything, they have no particular bias or goal other than giving clients complete satisfaction. Typically, however, they encourage surgery, since it is usually the most expensive option. Of course, a lifetime of hair additions can also be costly, but with surgery, the costs are paid immediately. These superstores typically suffer from all of the problems associated with surgical clinics, but because they offer hair additions and pharmaceutical treatments, they also have the problems associated with these branches of hair replacement.

Turnkey Operations

Once there was a time when marketing firms considered medical professions off-limits. Now, they specifically target doctors, especially those who are overburdened by managed care. The express intent of these marketing firms in the area of hair transplantation is to "help" physicians establish new practices literally overnight. The setup is so complete that all the doctor has to do is "turn the key" and open the door to a brand new hair-replacement office— hence, the term "turnkey" marketing.

Dr. Robert Leonard, past President of the International Society of Hair Restoration Surgery and hair-replacement specialist in Cranston, Rhode Island, recounts a personal experience with just such a marketing firm. He recalls, "I spoke with [a] marketing professional who, for a fee, [would have] provided before and after photos of patients [whose surgery was not performed by me], provided advice on marketing a hair-restoration practice, training for office staff to properly answer the phones, [and] training me (sic) how to do hair-transplant surgery. I asked him how he could do something like this. [The marketing man] responded that he observed the 'Masters,' and therefore, could walk me through my first few surgeries."

The marketer was literally offering Dr. Leonard a surgical hair-replacement franchise. Of course, this example represents the worst kind of abuse, but, unfortunately, it is not an isolated incident. And please don't think that we are lost in a haze of nostalgia for a kinder, gentler America. We realize that all doctors are not created equal, but the traditional safeguards for the patient have eroded to the degree that editorials on medical ethics appear in hair-replacement journals with a frequency that almost rivals the articles on surgical techniques.

Dr. Leonard is responsible for the "Medico-Legal" section of *The Hair Transplant Forum International.* It offers articles on the ethical decisions that surgeons make every day. Until recently, it was unheard of to include a section on ethics in a medical journal.

Is Training Always Sufficient?

Would you get on a plane knowing that the pilot's training consisted of a weekend seminar with a marketing consultant who had watched other pilots fly planes? Not unless someone held a gun to your head. Would you knowingly allow anyone to perform surgery on your head with the same kind of inadequate training? Of course not. Yet, in many cases, patients unwittingly allow surgeons who have had little or no training to operate on their heads.

Picture this scenario: Dr. X, who has been working in a hair-transplant clinic, feels that he has learned enough and is ready to open his own practice. He plans to leave in two weeks but has surgeries scheduled—one of which is yours—for the following two months. The clinic, or more specifically, its founding surgeon (who is also the CEO) now faces an ethical dilemma. Knowing that it will take several months to hire and train another doctor to replace Dr. X, does Dr. CEO inform you that Dr. X is leaving the clinic and that it will be necessary for you (and fifty other patients that were also scheduled for surgery with him) to have the surgery rescheduled? Or does he hire another doctor to step in immediately, regardless of his training, without notifying you? It may make perfect business sense for Dr. CEO to hire a replacement surgeon without informing the patients, but does it make professional sense?

Remember, this type of ethical dilemma can occur in any surgeon's office, large or small. However, the bigger the business, the greater the chance of such problems occurring.

Rationalizations

Certainly, if a doctor behaved in the unethical, unprincipled ways we have just described, you would avoid choosing him as your surgeon. Unfortunately, most doctors with such intentions aren't obvious, and they use subtle rationalizations to justify performing inappropriate procedures. These rationalizations typically fall into one of three major groups: 1) If I don't do it, someone else will; 2) The patient made me do it; and 3) I'm not my brother's keeper.

If I Don't Do It, Someone Else Will

Kenneth Bushwach, MD, the author of a textbook on surgical hair replacement, gave a lecture in 1996 about the long-term complications of scalp-reduction surgery. Because of these problems, he spoke of his intent to discontinue performing this type of surgery. At the end of the lecture, a noted surgeon stood and said, "Ken, you have an established cosmetic surgery practice in Kansas City. You can afford not to do these procedures. But if you lived here, where we have so many more plastic surgeons doing hair replacements, you wouldn't be able to turn patients away, because if you didn't do the procedures, someone else would. So, it might as well be me who does them, especially since I do them better than everyone else."

It is interesting to note that the offending doctor implicitly acknowledged that the procedures had inherent problems. Still, he rationalized that it was better to have a good surgeon perform a bad procedure rather than a bad surgeon. Although this may be true, it would be even better to have a good surgeon refuse to do a bad procedure regardless of the financial consequences to his practice.

The Patient Made Me Do It

If a woman went to a plastic surgeon and said that she'd like to have her ears attached backwards, would the surgeon do it just because she asked for it? Of course not. The surgeon would know full well that his reputation is at stake and he would never perform such an unnatural procedure. Yet somehow, when it comes to a man and his hair, many surgeons seem to abandon this very fundamental responsibility if it means losing a patient. They coyly claim, "The patient made me do it."

The rationalizing surgeon can even set up his patient as a convenient scapegoat by asking him, "What would you like? Where would you like your grafts?" Such questions should raise suspicions immediately. Can you imagine being wheeled into the operating room for open heart surgery and the surgeon leaning down to ask, "Bill, during today's surgery I will bypass the anterior descending artery, but as long as I'm in the neighborhood, do you want me to bypass the posterior coronary artery also?" The surgeon may ask for your cosmetic goals, but never for your "surgical plan."

I Am Not My Brother's Keeper

A distinguished hair surgeon approached Dr. Marritt at a surgical conference with one of his best-looking patients, a thirty-seven-year-old male. Dr. Marritt remarked, "This patient looks fabulous right now, but what about the fact that fifteen years from now, his head will look like a road map of exposed scars?" The doctor replied with all honesty, "I tell all my patients, nothing lasts forever. It's their decision. I'm not my brother's keeper."

Such utter disrespect for the patient is often revealed by the work performed. The ethical surgeon will make decisions that are in the best *long-term* interest of his patients.

COSMETIC HAIR ADDITIONS

The technology for making hair additions that look and feel real has made this a valuable option for anyone experiencing hair loss. Professionals working with cosmetic hair additions have always had more of a business focus than those involved in the other branches of hair replacement. This means that outrageous advertising and sales gimmicks occasionally make their way in the promotion of this business.

Swim, Shower, and Play?

Because it is true that you can get all the hair you want from hair additions, with certain exceptions that will be outlined in Chapter 4, the unethical hair-addition practitioner likes to use the "swim, shower, and play" tactic as an advertising tool. Almost every ad claims that you won't have to sacrifice any part of your busy active life. The hair addition, giving you all the hair you want, will not only remain perfectly in place at all times, it will also look and feel like human hair under any and all conditions. Some advertisers will also promise that because of some revolutionary attachment method, no cleaning or maintenance is needed. And, of course, the price is so low they may as well be giving them away.

Such pie-in-the-sky promises are pure fantasy. Hair additions, although improving all the time, are still detectable under certain circumstances, such as close inspection and extremely high winds. Plus, all hair additions need maintenance and cleaning on a regular basis. Some of the higher-end additions require that you purchase two so that while one is on your head, the other can be in the "shop," getting maintained. Moreover, even using human hair does not guarantee complete naturalness in feeling. Over time, human hair degrades from exposure to the elements. And although several new synthetic fibers feel totally natural, each one needs specific maintenance. In addition, the base of any hairpiece is made of a synthetic material that lies on the top of the head; and because it is not natural, it will not *feel* natural.

What are the consequences of believing the advertising hype? For the most part, you will be losing some money and, perhaps, a little dignity. However, some hair-addition attachment methods can cause permanent damage to the scalp if they are not handled correctly. The pros and cons of each type of attachment method are outlined in Chapter 4.

Hidden Costs

Many of the problems with surgical hair replacement are related to the withholding of information. The same is true of hair additions. What a hair-addition professional decides to tell you (or not tell you) will significantly affect the outcome of your purchase and your satisfaction with it. A lack of complete and proper information always leads to poor decisions.

One of the most common ways in which salesmen mislead customers is to hide costs in the fine print of a contract. Contracts should specify additional interest or payments, added maintenance charges, unusual fees for replacements or repairs, surcharges, and taxes. The person supplying your hair addition should be able to explain each and every cost that is stipulated in the contract. Ninety-nine percent of all hair-addition costs are based on three components: the hair itself, the base, and the method of attachment. (One exception—a new hair-addition process called Micro Point Link, discussed in Chapter 4—does not have a base.) Maintenance costs should also be factored in for normal wear and tear and the regular cleaning of additions. If you are charged for anything else, you're getting ripped off.

Regardless of their potential drawbacks, cosmetic hair additions, which continue to improve, represent a viable option for hair loss. Whether they are used as permanent solutions or temporary hair replacements prior to surgery, hair additions serve a valuable purpose.

PHARMACEUTICAL TREATMENTS

Like hair additions, the pharmaceutical treatment of hair loss also has a strong business focus. Most of the products that fall under this category are purposely designed to be used without a doctor's supervision, and, therefore, do not need FDA approval. As a result, the question of ethical boundaries in the area of pharmaceuticals is not clear. A lack of proper information is another major problem with this branch of the hair-replacement field.

Promises, Promises

Advertisements for pharmaceutical treatments usually promise the painless, quick, and easy return of all your lost hair, regardless of age or amount of hair loss. A full-page ad in *Sports Illustrated* for extra-strength Rogaine roared, "Gentlemen, Start Your Follicles!" What made this ad so ingenious is that nothing is stated overtly. No actual promise is made, but the implication is clear: Extra-strength Rogaine will jump-start your hair growth like high-octane fuel runs a racecar. That's a powerful message, but for the vast majority of men, it's also a false message, as you will soon learn in Chapter 5.

At this time, only Rogaine and Propecia have FDA approval for safety and efficacy to combat hair loss. More important, no other pharmaceutical treatment is backed by any legitimate scientifically approved testing to effectively reverse, stop, or even slow the balding process. It may be disheartening to hear this, but it is the truth.

With that said, currently, there is no product, pill, lotion, potion, or vitamin supplement—including Rogaine and Propecia—that can permanently reverse and cure male pattern baldness. Any pharmaceutical product claiming that it can is lying—no ifs, ands, or buts. Maybe someday there will be a drug that cures baldness, but at this time, all claims of a "cure" are false.

Snake Oils

As with most things in life, simple solutions rarely apply to complex situations. Most so-called pharmaceutical remedies—referred to as "snake oils"—are based on the assumption that male pattern baldness is caused by a biological deficiency or imbalance. This imbalance may seem plausible to the layperson, but, in actuality, has no sound basis in medical fact. These snake-oil products or treatments raise consumer hope by claiming to reverse hair loss by correcting the imbalance. This, however, is impossible. (Chapter 3 explains the actual cause of male pattern baldness.)

Before there were surgical clinics, salons typically sold snake-oil products or treatments that were designed to combat baldness. Thriving infomercials continue to present erroneous causes of hair loss to keep a number of ineffectual treatments alive, including the following:

• Avoiding hats or any objects that cover the head tightly.

- Standing on one's head periodically to increase blood flow to that area.

- Brushing the hair one hundred strokes daily for stimulation of the hair follicles.

- Washing with "special, scientifically formulated" shampoos and/or solutions—the exact ingredients of which are suspiciously kept secret.

- Using "special" topical creams or lotions to eliminate harmful bacteria from the scalp.

- Using electrical treatments to liquefy dead skin, dirt, and oil to dislodge them from the hair shaft.

- Taking daily vitamins and supplements.

- Using massage, heat lamps, and hot towels to dilate blood vessels in the head, which increases blood flow to the scalp.

As you can see, some of these "treatments" will cost the consumer nothing, while others can be very expensive. Most often, however, a combination of these snake-oil remedies is recommended. This usually means a trip to the hair salon for further unnecessary but costly treatments.

WHY IS THIS HAPPENING?

It is difficult to say with complete confidence why such bad business practices have invaded the field of hair replacement. It appears that a combination of greed and declining standards have conspired to help the invasion. Our nation's cultural shift from the 1970s to the 1980s also may have played a part. The 1970s was a decade of great change and social upheaval in America. It was a time of economic recession, the Vietnam War, the Watergate scandal, and such controversial court cases as Roe versus Wade. In stark contrast to the seventies, the eighties were a time of relative peace for Americans. The economy boomed. People felt rich and comfortable again.

Money to Spend, Money to Make

The seventies were over and there was money to be made. Expendable income became a new phrase in the American vocabulary. Luxury was in. The times had definitely changed for hair replacement. For cosmetic surgeons, it was the beginning of the financial golden age. While the intellectual elite was critical, saying that our obsession with appearance was damaging our culture, cosmetic surgery gained acceptance in ways never before imaginable. Once relegated to housewives trying to eliminate signs of aging, cosmetic surgery has expanded to include anyone and everyone, even men. But it wasn't only the cosmetic surgeons who benefited. After its announcement for Rogaine in 1988, Upjohn saw its stock triple. Also, the growth in technology for cosmetic hair additions was driven largely by an increased concern for natural appearance, which directly coincided with the overall acceptance of cosmetic surgery.

Estimates vary, but the total earnings of the field—including those from surgical hair rearrangement, cosmetic additions, and pharmaceutical treatments—have grown to more than a billion dollars per year. The lure of money is a formidable adversary, which certainly explains why unethical hair-addition providers and other salespeople affiliated with the field have no incentive to change their bad business practices. Unfortunately, money is partially the incentive for many doctors as well.

Doctors and Voluntary Compliance

Why do some doctors choose an unethical path? Perhaps it is because they have little incentive to change. In addition to the money they can make, the system of medicine is set up in such a way that it almost discourages doctors from changing. The concept of voluntary compliance means that it is the individual doctor alone who decides which new ideas he will or will not incorporate into his own private practice. This depends on a doctor's willingness to accept change and discard outmoded procedures. Accepting the scientific observations about male pattern baldness or a new surgical technique can be difficult even when supported by scientific evidence, because the evidence may be filtered through an emotional interaction between the patient and the doctor. Therefore, a doctor may prescribe inappropriate procedures because of his personal fear of aging, his own issues with baldness, or to maintain his position in the field of surgical hair rearrangement.

If, for example, a doctor develops a new surgical procedure, which, at the time, seems revolutionary, and becomes the world's leading authority in this technique, he may acquire academic prestige and wealth as a result. He will undoubtedly develop an emotional attachment to "his procedure." After years of building a reputation and an office empire, suddenly, long-term study and observation of his procedure reveals unsuspected complications. What seemed brilliant at one time is now exposed by objective scientific observation as not just mediocre but even damaging to the patient. The doctor faces a moral dilemma. Does he sacrifice his status and income in light of this new information? Who would want to start over at age fifty, learning new techniques, training new staff, and downsizing expenses and lifestyle?

More important, a surgeon in this position typically reacts from an emotional perspective and will not want to accept the death of a procedure that had once been so promising. Bruce Jafek, MD, a former department chair of Head and Neck Surgery at the University of Colorado said it like this, "In medicine, and surgery, you are always permitted to find new and interesting applications for an existing surgical procedure. You are never permitted to find fewer indications for an existing surgical procedure." And so, the hair-replacement field is flooded with many bad business habits and practices.

Declining Standards

It seems pretty straightforward to say that our culture has relaxed its standards. Morals, values, whatever you want to call them, have definitely changed. When the first ads for lawyers appeared on television, there was a large and loud debate throughout the medical industry. Although the consensus was that advertising was not acceptable for doctors, sure enough, some doctors started to advertise. Today, medical advertising is accepted as the norm. Many medical school graduates are not even aware that physicians were once prohibited from advertising. And so standards change.

Ultimately, however, it makes no difference why bad business practices have overtaken the field of hair replacement. It is only important to recognize that it has happened, and that you have to plan accordingly to avoid them.

THE LIGHT AT THE END OF THE TUNNEL

Is there a light at the end of the tunnel? The answer is a resounding yes. There are plenty of ethical doctors out there who do excellent work, enough so that every person reading this book will find one. Consider the motto of Robert Limmer, MD, a San Antonio dermatologist and hair-replacement surgeon: "The goal is what is best for the patient, not for the surgeon. Our role is to educate the patient on his options in a manner that reflects the highest levels of integrity as we all pledged to do when we became physicians." These words perfectly describe what to look for in anyone providing information about hair-replacement options, whether a doctor, salesman, or hair professional.

So, can you find a light at the end of the tunnel? Can you find an ethical doctor or hair-addition provider with the aid of this book? It is not only possible, but guaranteed. Through heightened awareness, you can avoid bad business practices and learn to view advertisements with a healthy dose of skepticism. Caution should always be your watchword, but never more so than when dealing with big business and its single-minded focus on the bottom line, which is rarely in your best medical interest.

CONCLUSION

We have outlined how the field of hair replacement has changed, but haven't discussed why this change has taken hold. In Chapter 2, "The Psychology of Baldness," we will discuss how negative business practices dovetail perfectly with personal fears and anxiety about hair loss. "Psychology?" you ask. Yes. And once you understand the origin of your fears, you will be less vulnerable, less likely to succumb to any emotionally manipulative practices used by unethical doctors or salesmen.

2

The Psychology
of Hair Loss

"It takes two to hear the truth—one to speak and another to hear."

—HENRY DAVID THOREAU, AMERICAN PHILOSOPHER

hapter 1 gave you some insight into the business of hair replacement and how some doctors and hair providers may not be as straightforward as you might like to think they are. The best way to fully protect yourself is through knowledge—to become aware of the facts and understand how and why you may be vulnerable. Unfortunately, there is one thing that often stands in the way of most people gaining this knowledge—their emotions.

This chapter looks at the reactions you are likely to have regarding hair loss, and helps you understand them. It explains how and why this is a particularly vulnerable time for you—a time during which it is all too easy to make unwise decisions. It then presents guidelines for handling your emotions in a constructive way, which will allow you to gain the knowledge you need to make the best and most satisfying hair-replacement choices.

FIRST THE COUCH, THEN THE TABLE

At this point in the book, you may be wondering, "Aren't we supposed to be talking about hair?" Well, we *are* talking about hair, we're just approaching it from a different angle. Many men and women are vulnerable because hair loss has specific psychological and emotional symptoms that can result in harmful behavior. It's important to understand these symptoms to insure the long-term health and safety of your head. Therefore, before you get to lie down on the operating table or choose another way to manage your hair loss, you must first lie down on the psychoanalyst's couch—figuratively speaking—in order to understand the psychology of baldness as it relates to you.

So how will understanding the psychology of baldness help treat your hair loss? As a prospective hair-treatment consumer, you can never understand the outside of your head (your hair loss), until you first understand the inside of your head (the emotional reaction to your hair loss). This understanding will help you to think logically, thereby leading you to the best doctor or hair provider, who will then propose the most appropriate surgical technique or hair addition for you.

COMMON MALE REACTIONS TO HAIR LOSS

Hair loss can produce a host of reactions, including panic, anger, denial, and jealousy. While most men will face some or all of these reactions, they will experience them differently.

Panic

Fueled by fear and desperation, many men panic at the sight of their thinning hair. Specifically, this triggers masculinity issues. Many worry: Will women find me unattractive? Will I look too old to get that promotion at work? Will people consider me "over the hill?" and on and on . . . Hair loss can and often does evoke the feeling that life as you know it is over. In this respect, baldness is perceived as a matter of life and death.

Take the example of Harold Brodkey, whose story appeared in *The New Yorker* magazine. The sixty-nine-year-old went to the doctor for a routine physical and some lab tests. When he returned for the results a week later, his doctor told him that he had a terminal illness. After letting the truth of the statement soak in for a moment, Harold's first words were, "Look, it's only death. It's not like losing your hair." Apparently, the saying "Time heals all wounds" doesn't always heal the wound of male pattern baldness—at least not in this case. Of course, rationally, Mr. Brodkey knew the difference between death and the death of hair follicles. Emotionally, however, he associated the loss of his hair with a fate worse than death.

Denial

Denial plays a role in almost every reaction and emotion that a man feels about his hair loss. Men want to deny everything—that they are losing their hair, that they find it upsetting, and that they cannot handle it emotionally. Recognizing and coping with denial, which is a lie to oneself, is the most important and yet the most difficult part of understanding the psychology of baldness. How can you find the truth if you're starting with a lie? Denial prevents an accurate assessment of the condition of baldness and its realistic treatment options; and this can lead to poor treatment choices. Why do you think that close to a billion dollars is spent on bogus baldness cures every year?

Humiliation

Men often complain to us that their hair loss has caused them to become a joke among their friends. Many claim that they first realized they were balding when their "best friend" announced it in the locker room, causing other guys to take notice and then start taunting. Feeling panicked, the person experiencing hair loss finds himself in a defensive position. He's also in a bind. If he reacts to the teasing with anything other than mute acceptance, he risks being perceived as less than a man, which is exactly how he may already feel due to his thinning hair. So, the best of his seemingly bad options is to take the teasing "like a man" without comment.

The public nature of male confrontation only makes a difficult situation worse, and almost always produces feelings of severe humiliation. These feelings can be intense, and because facing them can be painful, avoidance (denial) is sometimes the preferred option.

On the day of his surgery, a patient of Dr. Marritt brought along his wife. To show her what would be done during the procedure, Dr. Marritt unexpectedly called the woman from the waiting room into the operating room. What ensued was an awkward period of silence between the man and his wife as they stared uncomfortably at each other. Afterward, she told Dr. Marritt that in sixteen years of marriage, she had never seen her husband's bald head exposed. He was so ashamed of his baldness and so fearful of letting his wife see it that he had taken great pains to hide it. He would get up at five in the morning to shower and dress before she got out of bed. It was an unspoken rule that she was not allowed in the bathroom while he was dressing and blow-drying his hair.

How humiliated this man must have been, feeling the need to hide his baldness from his own wife. She was the one person who vowed to love him in sickness and in health, for richer or poorer, but apparently (he feared), not through baldness.

Desperation

After living with the humiliation of hair loss, many men become desperate to decrease their emotional pain, which often triggers impulsive behavior. Here's an example. Before coming to our office, a patient had met with a "hair specialist," who told him that his hair loss was caused by the lack of humidity in his hometown. It was recommended that he buy a head steamer. Desperate to "cure" his baldness, the patient actually moved to Florida because of its humid climate. After living a short time in this new location, not only was he still bald, he was sweaty, too! It didn't take long for him to realize that losing hair had little to do with humidity.

Fixation

The confrontational teasing discussed earlier can also provoke fixation, which often co-exists with desperation. Fixation is a psychological condition often caused by some overwhelming trauma, like the death of a loved one or a nasty divorce. If unable to integrate the psychic repercussions of the trauma, a person may become fixated or stuck in his emotional development by harboring all the feelings associated with that trauma, sometimes for years after the event.

To further explain, consider forty-five-year-old Stewart, who visited our office several years ago. He was completely bald in the back of his head with only a few hairs growing in the front. When Dr. Harris began to draw a hairline on the front of his head during the consultation, Stewart demanded that all of the grafts be placed in the back of his head. Dr. Harris then took him to the mirror and showed him that by covering only the back area, there wouldn't be any change in his facial appearance.

After further discussion, Stewart revealed that he wanted the hair transplanted in that area because of something that had happened years ago. A "friend" in his college gym class had made a comment regarding the spreading monk's spot on the back of Stewart's head. The comment quickly escalated into severe teasing, and from that point on, Stewart became fixated on that area of his baldness. It was as if an emotional branding iron had burned that spot with a "B for Bald." Regardless of how bald he had become over the rest of his head, hair loss meant only one thing to him—the bald spot on the back of his head.

Subconscious Jealousy

Typically, bald men experience jealousy because they desperately covet what their non-bald brothers have. Terry Bradshaw, the Pittsburgh Steelers' famed quarterback of the seventies, while acting as color commentator for Super Bowl XXIII, called John Elway of the Denver Broncos spoiled, overpaid, and overrated as a quarterback. Elway calmly responded by saying that Bradshaw was just jealous because the salaries were so much lower when he played. Nine years later in 1998's Super Bowl XXXII, John Elway and the Broncos emerged victorious. Once again, Terry Bradshaw was the color commentator for the event. At one point during the game, Bradshaw reluctantly admitted that he *was* jealous of Elway's salary... *and* of Elway's hair.

Feelings of Isolation

Even though most men who are balding share the same feelings, each man, ironically, tends to feel completely alone. Please remember that you are *not* alone. For nearly three decades, we have spoken to thousands of men—every size, shape, and color—about their hair loss. They all have fears, desires, and needs. Unfortunately, many men also felt constrained and isolated by social pressures dictating that they shouldn't display such feelings, much less concern over their appearance. Men often feel that they must hold in their emotions and appear stoic and strong; showing their feelings is considered a sign of weakness. Unfortunately, these efforts to appear strong serve only to isolate them from one another.

Conversely, women don't have such emotional constraints. They tend to be more comfortable in expressing their feelings and maintaining their beauty by whatever means necessary. Comedienne Phyllis Diller openly and shamelessly talked and even joked about her facelifts for years. But how is it possible for men to get hair, much less get hair appropriately, without admitting that they want it?

UNDERSTANDING YOUR REACTIONS

After many years of talking to patients, it is clear that there are several major reasons for the range of feelings that men experience over hair loss. While these may not be the only reasons, the following discussions may help shed light on your own reactions to hair loss.

Society's Values

Hair has fascinated humans since the beginning of time. Different from the hair of most other mammals, human hair is extremely visible as an identifying trait. As a result, hair has assumed an extremely symbolic role in human life, defining political, social, religious, sexual, and economic status.

In 1991, a man from the Neolithic Age was found frozen in a glacier near the Austrian-Italian border. Interestingly, this man, who was believed to be around 5,300 years old, had hair that was cut in a very neat, precise style. He must have considered the appearance of his hair important.

But styles come and go. During the 1700s, both men and women of the upper classes wore wigs. Some of these hairpieces were very elaborate, and included such ornamentation as birdcages (complete with live birds), small models of famous buildings, and other intricate decorations. It was simply the fashion. Today, however, no prominent businessman—the "aristocrat" of our times—would wear a wig adorned with anything. It's just not the trend. What's important to understand is that values change, and while cultures the world over have their individual beliefs and rules concerning appropriate hairstyles, these beliefs are always changing.

Currently, American culture places a great deal of value on youth, and, therefore, on a youthful appearance. Because a full head of hair is associated with being young, it is considered a good thing. Unfortunately, on the flip side, balding is associated with aging. The fact, of course, is that intrinsically, hair or the lack of it is neither good nor bad. No one in any field of scientific study has served up a plausible reason why humans even have hair in the first place. The problem is only that our society values a full head of hair—at least for the moment. So remember that while you are experiencing real feelings, part of their intensity is nothing more than a response to the subjective beliefs of society.

It's Not the Hair, It's the Loss

Some of the most stressful situations in life, such as the death of a loved one, the loss of a job, or the diagnosis of a life-threatening illness, will elicit predictable feelings of sadness, fear, anger, frustration, and panic. Although initially these stressful situations may appear different from one another, a second look reveals a common denominator—loss. The problem with hair loss isn't really the lack of hair, but the emotional response to the loss.

Along with losing your hair, you are also losing the dream of youth, mostly because baldness makes one look older. Hair loss has always been associated with aging (even the baldest man at age sixty had hair at sixteen). That's just the way male pattern baldness works. It is a condition of advancing age. Thoughts of getting older, however, eventually trigger thoughts of death, which we spend the majority of our lives trying to avoid. For most men, the unconscious association regarding hair loss is:

Loss of hair = Loss of youth = Inevitable aging = Death

These associative links have a domino effect. Once the mind has completed the chain, man's most basic instinct—survival—

takes over immediately. It mobilizes a combination of desperation and denial. And although everyone knows that "No one lives forever," no one wants to believe it. So people comfort themselves by saying, "I'm not *that* bald; I'm still young." But eventually, progressive baldness becomes difficult to ignore because of its high visibility. This is why men may cover their heads with hats or begin parting their hair a bit lower than they should—anything not to see their hair loss. Out of sight, out of mind. And there's nothing wrong with a little denial. But be careful. A little denial can quickly become a lot of denial. And it often does.

Baldness Makes You Look Different

Unlike other visible signs of aging, such as wrinkles or a sagging chin, which tend to creep up slowly over many years, baldness can strike suddenly, swiftly, and extensively. One patient who came to our office had started to lose his hair at age nineteen. By twenty-three, he had little more than a horseshoe of hair around the perimeter of his head. His youthful appearance had disappeared as he was transformed into a replica of his father, seemingly in the blink of an eye. He said of his hair loss, "I look twenty-five from the eyes down, and sixty from the eyebrows up." Not surprisingly, he could not accept the difference between his self-image and his actual appearance.

Part of the difficulty in accepting his appearance was due to the high visibility of baldness as a sign of aging—much more so than crow's feet or a sagging chin. Let's compare. Crow's feet and sagging chins are usually measured in millimeters; the results of which, while not welcome, are not dramatic enough to make a twenty-five year old suddenly look like his grandfather. And perhaps more important is the fact that wrinkles, by and large, are tolerated in men. Men who have lined faces are sometimes thought of as rugged or distinguished. In stark contrast to such "rugged" wrinkles, baldness can be measured in square inches, visible even from across a crowded room. Such a dramatic and extensive change in appearance serves only to increase the sense of loss of a familiar self-image, making it more difficult to accept.

The difference between self-image and reality may also exist for the man who has just lost his first few hairs. Although he may still have almost all of his hair, initial panic may cause him to imagine himself looking like a billiard ball by next week. The anticipated loss of his youthful self-image can consume him with fear. Either way, whether anticipated or actual, a psychological conflict arises from a perceived difference between the picture in the mind and the picture in the mirror. For the young man who balds quickly, the change in appearance is most dramatic and alarming. Of course, in the minds of all men, no time is considered a good time to bald.

The Influence of Testosterone

Testosterone is a hormone that serves an important biochemical function within the male body. In addition to giving men their competitiveness and sexual drive, testosterone causes them to become assertive, mark their territory, and take action—traits that typically define "maleness." But lose one hair and this same "maleness" may prompt one to act too quickly. Remember the man we discussed earlier in the chapter who moved to Florida? A man's very nature may interfere with his ability to act calmly and rationally while handling the emotional repercussions of hair loss.

WHAT SHOULD YOU DO?

Can you help yourself deal with these unsettling emotions? Although you may never be pleased by the fact that you are losing your hair, there are several steps you can take to help overcome your heightened emotional state. Begin with an honest look at what you expect to achieve with hair replacement—what are your goals? Try to verbalize your feelings—your pain, fears, and frustrations—with someone you trust. Also, allow yourself some time to grieve over your hair loss. Finally, do your homework and become aware of all of your options. These few steps, which are detailed in the following discussion, will help you to calmly assess both the reality of your situation and your options.

Understand Your Goals

There are two ultimate goals you can hope to achieve with hair replacement—getting hair and feeling better about yourself. Most men think that getting hair is more important, and by achieving that goal, they will automatically feel better. While the lucky man may succeed by approaching the situation from such a perspective, most men will fail. Remember, your unhappiness with hair loss is not caused only by the simple loss of your hair, but with other issues—lost youth, changing self-image, and damaged self-esteem. As mentioned before, these issues, if left unresolved, often become unconscious motivations that push you into making unwise or premature decisions. As a result, the most important goal for the man experiencing hair loss is to confront these issues and attempt to work through them—to find a way to feel better about himself before he starts the search for hair.

But many men will argue, "Exactly how can I feel better about myself if I'm unhappy about my hair loss?" The idea is to separate the hair loss from your self-esteem. Clearly, your worth—your competence as a man and your ability to be a good person, for instance—is not dependent on your hairline. Many men, nevertheless, make such associations whether they admit it or not, and sometimes, whether they know it or not. The point is to first realize that you may be making such destructive associations, and then realign the way you think. By allowing yourself to go through a grieving process and by talking out your feelings, you may actually discover that you can be happy *without* a full head of hair. If not, at least you'll be ready to calmly review your hair-replacement options, and then choose an approach that is best for you.

Talk to Someone

Talk to your spouse, your brother, your priest—anyone you can trust to listen and understand your frustration and pain. If you have a close friend who has lost his hair, broach the topic with him (if you feel comfortable doing so). His reaction to hair loss may be different from yours, and a frank conversation may give you a new perspective. Most important, discuss your feelings with your doctor or a qualified hair provider before committing to any procedures.

Our experience has shown that many patients have difficulty talking at first. Caught up in the agony of panic and desperation, most feel that talking is a waste of time. Some consider it to be a sign of weakness and an invitation to more humiliation. Instead of viewing talking as a waste of time, money, and emotional energy, think of it as prevention. By talking about your feelings, understanding them, and acknowledging them, you can transform your pressing "need" to get hair into a simple and straightforward desire. If you don't "need" to get hair, then you can wait; you know you have time. You can research your options calmly, and avoid being misled and deceived.

Sure you may want hair, but you won't need it to bolster your self-esteem. You'll probably never like your baldness, but talking about it will help you accept it. And accepting your hair loss will help make you the perfect candidate for hair replacement.

Allow Yourself to Grieve

As discussed earlier in this chapter, one cause of your emotional reaction stems from the sadness you feel over your loss. Therefore, it is vital that you allow yourself time to grieve. Grieving involves introspection, talking, thinking, feeling, crying, cursing, laughing, and screaming in no particular order, and for no particular period of time. It will take as long as it takes, but when it's over, it's over.

Denial and all of the other emotions you may be feeling have a potentially dangerous effect on your decision-making process. You may rush to do "something," which means you are thinking short-term—looking for instant gratification. Nonetheless, it's only natural to think such short-term, misguided thoughts when you are constantly bombarded with manipulative advertising that encourages you to act impulsively and "Just do it!" Doing, or acting out, is really an attempt to resolve painful feelings with a quick fix. Sadly, such attempts don't work.

Many men with hair loss rush for the quick fix because they cannot imagine anything in the world that's worse than being bald, but they have limited imaginations. Far worse is developing an infection from having a hairpiece sutured to your head. Far worse is having an alopecia-reduction scar running across the back of your head. Far worse is having poorly transplanted hair grafts that result in plugginess, which may ultimately force you to wear a hair addition.

The grieving process and the acceptance of hair loss will help you avoid such catastrophes. If you don't "need" hair, but merely "want" it, you will be better prepared to hear the truth about what you can realistically do to get it. For any hair-replacement option, there must be an acceptance of some type of compromise. The exact nature of the compromises and the reasons why you must accept them will be fully discussed in Chapter 8, "Decisions, Decisions."

Examine Your Options

There are very strict rules governing how to treat hair loss safely and permanently. Because of this, the amount of hair most men are able to get is restricted, so the vast majority get less hair than they want. Therefore, it is extremely important to think long and hard before making treatment decisions. The only way to ensure the long-term safety of your head is through the calm and thorough examination of your options and the clear knowledge of the various procedures and their limitations. These procedures will be detailed later in the book.

TOUGH LOVE

Maybe we've been a bit tough on you in this chapter, but we feel that it is necessary to break through your subconscious defenses of denial and desperation. These concepts are troublesome and especially difficult when understanding them ultimately means accepting compromise. Once you have truly grieved over the death of your hair, it will be easier for you to accept the fact that you cannot have it all back. This acceptance will make a significant difference in the hair-replacement choice you make.

CONCLUSION

Now that we have discussed the inside of your head, it's time to move on to the outside. Chapter 3 explains what does and what does not cause baldness. This information will help you begin the process of outlining what you can do to realistically, safely, and permanently deal with your hair loss.

3

The Causes
of Hair Loss

"Ours is an age in which partial truths are tirelessly transformed into
total falsehoods and then acclaimed as revolutionary revelations."

—THOMAS SZASZ, WRITER

Ever since Hippocrates recorded the first scientific observation
regarding the causes of baldness, countless scientists and doctors have also made sound observations—and yet many pro-
ceeded to ignore the truth and either create or embrace false
theories. In fact, the medical community at large did not widely
accept the realities of hair loss until well into the second half of the
twentieth century.

In 1955, Norman Orentreich, MD, a noted New York City dermatologist specializing in hair-loss research, wrote his original
watershed paper on grafting and baldness but had difficulty publishing it. The review committees and editorial staffs of the major
journals could not and would not believe Orentreich's findings,
so they rejected his article. Finally, four years later in 1959, a little-
known journal called *The Annals of the New York Academy of Sciences*
agreed to publish his paper. In it, Orentreich's groundbreaking
experiment, which is discussed later in this chapter, dispelled
many myths about the causes of baldness.

Although the actual causes of baldness are widely known and
accepted in the scientific community today, many people still
choose to believe folklore, fiction, and fantasies. This is demonstrated by the number of bogus cures that continue to flood the

market. This chapter is designed to help set everything straight. First, it provides basic information about the anatomy and life cycle of the hair follicle. Then it debunks the common myths regarding hair loss, and follows with a detailed discussion of the true causes of baldness.

HAIR BASICS

To understand hair loss, it is important to have knowledge of hair basics, including the structure of hair and its life cycle, the balding process, and the normal maturation of the hairline.

The Structure of Hair

Every hair on your body grows from a small pouch-like structure in your skin called a *follicle*. Hair follicles range in size from 3 to 4 millimeters in length and each produces a hair, which can be one of several types. *Terminal* hairs are those that people consider their "normal" hair. Terminal hair continues to grow well after it's cut, and has color and texture that is similar to the hair found in areas of the scalp without hair loss. *Vellus* hairs are very thin and fine, soft in texture, and lighter in color than terminal hairs. They are often found at the very front of the hairline or in the space between a bald and hair-bearing area. *Intermediate* hairs tend to be somewhat thinner, softer, shorter, and lighter in color than terminal hairs, but not quite vellus-like. In fact, intermediate hairs come from follicles that are in transition and will eventually produce a vellus hair. This will be explained shortly in the discussion on the balding process.

The *hair follicle,* as seen in Figure 3.1 on page 39 is a club-shaped structure that extends from the upper layer of skin called the *epidermis* to the deeper middle layer called the *dermis*. The main portion of the follicle is composed of seven different and interconnecting layers. The three main layers include the outer root sheath, the inner root sheath, and the hair shaft. The *outer root sheath* surrounds the follicle in the dermis, and then blends into the epidermis on the surface of the skin. As the outer root sheath blends with the skin, it forms a pore, from which the hair exits the skin. The middle layer of the follicle is part of the structure that holds the

FIGURE 3.1. THE HAIR FOLLICLE

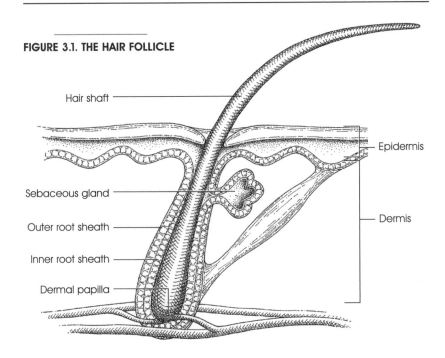

Hair shaft

Epidermis

Sebaceous gland

Dermis

Outer root sheath

Inner root sheath

Dermal papilla

hair in place. Part of the *inner root sheath* is made of an overlapping layer of cells that interlocks with the hair shaft, whose cells layer in the opposite direction. The meshing of the two layers keeps the hair anchored in the skin while allowing it to grow. The *hair shaft* is the part of the hair that you can see and comb.

The lower portion of the follicle widens into a region called the *bulb*. The bulb contains cells that determine the width of the fully grown hair. A small opening at the base of the bulb contains a group of specialized cells called the *dermal papilla.* The growth center of the hair extends from the dermal papilla all the way up to the region of the follicle near the skin's surface, where the *sebaceous glands* are attached. It is believed that the dermal papilla's main function is to regulate hair growth. Interestingly, if the dermal papilla is removed, which sometimes happens during a hair transplant, the hair follicle is capable of regrowing a hair, although the growth will be delayed. Each sebaceous gland secretes oil through the pore and along the hair shaft.

Now that you know the basic structure of hair, it's important to understand its life cycle.

The Life Cycle of Hair

Each hair follicle goes through a repeating growth cycle, which is made up of three phases—the *anagen* or growth phase, the *catagen* or transitional phase, and the *telogen* or resting phase. Some follicles also go through an *exogen* or "hairless" telogen phase.

A follicle in the anagen phase is actively producing a hair. At any given time, about 85 percent of the hairs on one's head are in this phase, which lasts from two to six years.

After completing the anagen phase, the follicle goes into the catagen phase, which lasts from one to two weeks. It is during this transitional phase that the follicle ceases to produce hair. The follicle itself shortens and separates from the dermal papilla.

The telogen phase is characterized by the continued shrinkage of the follicle and its migration toward the skin's surface. During this phase, which usually lasts five to six weeks, the hair may be shed during washing or brushing, or pushed out by a new hair as the follicle enters a new anagen growth phase. If, however, the hair falls out before a new anagen phase has begun, the follicle is considered to be in exogen. In some follicles, this period can last up to twelve months.

The Balding Process

Most people think that the balding process involves simply losing hairs from the head; however, it actually involves two simultaneous processes. First, the anagen growth phase becomes progressively shorter, and second, the follicle itself begins to shrink. The cause of these changes will be discussed in detail later in this chapter. These transformations occur over the course of several generations of the hair growth cycle, eventually resulting in a hair that is shorter, thinner, and with less pigment. This gradual reduction in the length of the anagen phase, along with a progressively shrinking follicle, are what cause a terminal hair's transition to an intermediate hair, and then eventually to a vellus hair.

The Mature Hairline

As you grow from child to adult, your hairline changes. During the normal male maturation process, the hairline on a prepubescent forehead naturally recedes approximately 2 centimeters during puberty. The hair may also thin slightly—usually due to a reduction in the diameter of individual hairs. This is considered the mature hairline. From this point on, any hair loss beyond the mature hairline is considered *male pattern baldness.*

About 80 percent of females will develop hairline recessions in the temple area, at times, even severe. Unlike men, most women will maintain the hairline at the center region of their forehead.

MYTHS ABOUT THE CAUSES OF BALDNESS

We have heard so many myths about the causes of baldness that it is sometimes difficult to know where to start discrediting them. People will blame anything. (Remember the outrageous myth in Chapter 2 that blamed lack of humidity for baldness?) Since it's impossible to cover every misconception regarding hair loss, we will identify the most common ones.

Mental Stress and Physical Trauma

It is a common yet mistaken belief that physical trauma and mental stress, including anguish and fear, cause hair loss. Patients are constantly telling us that they didn't start balding until a daughter started dating, or they began feeling the pressure of financial strain, or they were going through a divorce. Still others swear that their hair loss began after receiving some type of physical blow or trauma to the head, typically the result of an accident. Are these reasons valid? No. Although stress can speed up hair loss, especially in women, it is not the root cause.

From a psychological standpoint, what these people believe has caused their hair loss is actually a delayed reaction to a process that had already begun. In other words, their hair began to thin *before* the accident or *before* their daughter started dating. Only afterwards, in a state of heightened awareness from the trauma or stress, did they start to focus on their thinning hair—and this is a typical psychological reaction.

The Faulty Freeway System

The myth we refer to as the "faulty freeway system" is one of the most prevalent misconceptions for hair loss, and one that is still taught in some barber and beauty schools. This theory is based on the observation that there is less blood flow to the very top of the head compared to the lower portions of the scalp. Supposedly, because of this circulatory flaw—the faulty freeway system—the hair follicles are deprived of necessary nutrients, allowing toxins to accumulate. Subsequently, the hair starves and falls out. The theory further proposes that wearing a hat or headgear also restricts circulation to the head, worsening the already decreased supply of blood. The result? Hair loss. So what's wrong with this theory? Plenty.

The blood supply to the scalp is provided by branches of the left and right carotid arteries, which extend upward from the heart, curve around the ears, and continue upward like the branches of a tree to the very top of the head. Therefore, if the circulatory system determined baldness, it would follow that *all* men and *all* women would begin to bald in a center line that starts at the top of the head, runs to the frontal hairline, and gradually widens toward the ears. Obviously, this is not what happens. On the contrary, the earliest sign of baldness for the majority of men is thinning hair in the *temporal zone*—the area just above the temples—where the blood supply is greater than it is at the top of the head. Hair loss here forms *temporal* or *lateral recessions,* triangular or v-shaped balding spots, as seen in Figure 3.2 below.

There are other facts that refute the proposed connection between the circulatory system and hair loss. For instance, as people approach middle age—thirty-five to fifty-five—they tend to develop unwanted hair growth in their ears and nostrils, and on

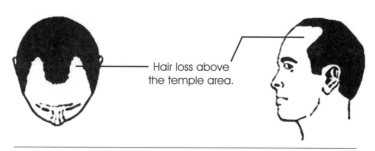

Hair loss above
the temple area.

FIGURE 3.2. V-SHAPED TEMPORAL (LATERAL) RECESSIONS

their eyebrows. Is it possible that suddenly, without noticeable cause, the blood supply to the ears, nose, and eyebrows increases in all middle-aged men? Not likely.

One final blow to the reduced blood supply theory is seen in Dr. Orentreich's 1955 experiment. He took a 4-millimeter hair-bearing graft with intact follicles from the back of a patient's head, as well as a 4-millimeter bald graft from the top of the same patient's head where extensive hair loss had occurred. Then Dr. Orentreich switched the two grafts, putting the hair-bearing graft in the hole left by the bald graft and vice versa. Over a period of several months, the "hairy" graft flourished in the vast space of baldness, and the bald one remained naked in the sea of hair that surrounded it. If blood supply affects hair loss and/or growth, the hair would have fallen out of the graft that was placed in the bald area. Conversely, the bald graft would have grown hair.

Cleanliness Is Next to Hairiness

According to this theory, a fatal cocktail of excess oil, air pollutants, sebum, and dead cells becomes lodged around the hair shaft, choking the hair and rendering it incapable of growth. The obvious question then is, "Why does the hair on the other areas of the head—specifically the sides and back—continue to flourish?" The *trichologist*, or hair-clinic expert, may explain that these hairs grow in a downward direction, causing the deadly accumulation to slide down the hairs away from the shaft and follicle, thus protecting the hair. But this is simply not true.

The theory that hair loss is caused by a dirty scalp fails to account for both the legions of clean yet bald men, and the multitudes of slovenly males with grimy yet full heads of hair. Populations in countries where the opportunity and resources for personal hygiene are scarce would experience rapid hair loss in both male and female inhabitants. Of course, nothing is further from the truth. Furthermore, if the whole scalp is dirty, wouldn't the entire scalp bald at the same time?

Developing good scalp and hair hygiene, including daily shampooing, is a desirable grooming habit that will make your existing hair more attractive. However, it will neither prevent hair fallout nor cause it to regrow.

You Are What You Eat

The "you are what you eat" or "vitamin supplement" theory proposes that the hair follicles of men who experience hair loss are deprived of essential nutrients, causing the follicles to die. This theory focuses on dietary supplements of vitamins and trace minerals, such as zinc, the amino acid cystine, and the B-complex vitamin biotin, as the best means of combating baldness.

Misleading advertisements will say that laboratory research has shown that hair, which is composed primarily of protein, must be fed certain vitamins, minerals, and amino acids for growth. Typically, the argument states that the average American's diet is sorely lacking in these critical nutrients; therefore, replacing them will combat hair loss.

Is it possible for a nutritional deficiency to cause balding? Yes, but it must be so severe that the person is literally dying from lack of food. Occasional deficiencies found in the average healthy person, such as short-term low levels of magnesium or zinc, are not the same as acute clinical starvation. Furthermore, clinical starvation does not and cannot cause hair loss in the patterns recognized as common male pattern baldness. Instead, it causes general or diffuse hair loss over the entire scalp. Moreover, hair loss is never the only symptom of clinical malnutrition, and it is usually one of the last. Other symptoms include but are not limited to conditions or diseases of the internal organs, teeth, gums, skin, and nails. Therefore, if you have diffuse unpatterned hair loss, but no other signs of acute clinical starvation, it is safe to assume that a nutritional deficiency is not the cause.

Learning From the Eskimos

Perhaps the Eskimos provide the best example of a culture that negates the common baldness myths. Eskimo males rarely wash their hair and wear hats most of the time. They also frequently apply whale and fish oils to their hair for sheen, which is considered pleasing in their culture. In addition, their restricted diet, consisting mostly of protein and fat, lacks the variety of foods to qualify as balanced.

Subject to every mythic cause of baldness, the Eskimo male is a victim of poor circulation due to cold temperature, further decreased blood supply resulting from the wearing of hats, a sebum-clogged scalp, and a diet that is lacking in essential vitamins—all of which, according to the myths, should produce an unusually high rate of baldness. However, like others with similar racial characteristics, the Eskimos have much less chance of experiencing baldness than the average Caucasian male.

THE TRUE CAUSES OF BALDNESS

Now that we have discussed the myths regarding baldness, it's time for the truth. There are numerous types of hair loss, each with its own cause and characterized by its own pattern or presentation. We will discuss each in turn, beginning with androgenetic alopecia, the type that affects the majority of men and some women.

Androgenetic Alopecia

Androgenetic alopecia is perhaps best known as common male pattern baldness. *Alopecia* is the Greek word for baldness, and *androgenetic* includes the words *androgens* (male hormones) and *genetic* (genes). However, heredity and hormones are only two of the three main components that cause common baldness. The third is time. Remove any one of these factors and you will not go bald.

First, let's take a closer look at each of these aspects in the development of androgenetic alopecia. Then we'll discuss the differences in this condition between males and females.

Heredity

As implied in the word andro*genetic*, genes are an important difference between the individual who goes bald and the one who doesn't. A person must first have the inherited tendency to bald before time and hormones can play their respective roles.

For all that we know about the inheritance of baldness, unfortunately, we don't know everything. We do not understand why some follicles are programmed to die at certain times over the course of one's life in a patterned manner. We don't know why a person who has parents with strong histories of baldness on both the maternal and paternal sides may not develop baldness. And we don't understand why this same person can have a son who then develops the balding characteristics of his grandfather or his grandmother's brothers.

We don't know why some men with family histories of extensive hair loss bald only slightly; nor do we know why men bald at varying rates or start losing their hair at different times. And we don't know why some members of a family develop extensive baldness while others do not—we have often heard the complaint, "My brother is ten years older than I am, but I'm already twice as bald as he is!"

Male Hormones

Hormones play many roles in the chemical processes of the body. Androgens and estrogens are the hormones specifically responsible for the development of typical sex-related traits. For the purposes of this discussion, only two androgens concern us: *testosterone* and its first cousin *dihydrotestosterone* (DHT). Although quite similar in their biochemical structure, testosterone and DHT have distinctly different effects on the body. Testosterone deepens the voice, builds muscle mass, and promotes hair growth under the arms and in the pubic area. Hair growth on the face and body, acne, prostate enlargement, and male pattern baldness are all under the control of DHT.

Although DHT is directly responsible for male pattern baldness, testosterone plays an integral role in the process. In the absence of testosterone, the body cannot make DHT, and without DHT, male pattern baldness cannot occur. Although the condition is called male pattern baldness, some women do experience hair loss in the same patterns as men with subtle variations. This will be discussed shortly.

In the human body, biochemical reactions do not take place spontaneously. They require the assistance of protein molecules called enzymes. In order for the body to make DHT, it must have both testosterone and the enzyme *5 alpha-reductase* (5αR). This enzyme is responsible for converting testosterone to DHT. It is the presence of DHT in the hair follicle that activates baldness. However, it is not understood how DHT can trigger hair loss on the head and at the same time cause hair to grow on the face.

The proof that DHT is directly responsible for causing hair loss came in 1975, when it was discovered that some male and female members of a family from the Dominican Republic had a genetic alteration that prevented their bodies from making 5αR. Although they had normal testosterone levels, they were not able to make DHT. All the women with this genetic change appeared entirely normal. The men did not bald at all.

Time

Time is the third and final factor that is necessary to cause baldness. Simply put—baldness is a condition of advancing age. It takes time for the genetically inherited balding tendency to manifest itself.

Differences Between the Sexes

Men and women with androgenetic alopecia may have hair-loss patterns that are similar, that is, both experience thinning in front or on top of the head. But in spite of this similarity, there are obvious differences in the balding patterns between the sexes. Men tend to lose hair in the frontal hairline, the temple areas, and the *crown*—the top or highest part of the head (where one would wear a crown). This process can result in the complete loss of hair in these areas. Women, on the other hand, tend to retain their frontal hairlines, and any thinning that may occur often takes place in the *forelock area*—the zone behind the frontal hairline and on top of the scalp. It is rare for women to lose all the hair in any thinning area. Also, women typically do not have as much recession near the temples as men do. However, by age sixty, 50 percent of women have significant recessions in this area. Another major difference is that women may also have significant thinning of the fringe area, while most men do not.

The Ludwig Chart on page 49 illustrates the typical progressive stages of thinning hair from female pattern baldness. The Norwood Classification Chart on pages 50 to 51 displays the typical hair-loss patterns experienced by males.

Unlike females, who tend to lose their hair in the same general area and in a similar fashion, males can experience differing patterns of loss, as seen in the Norwood Chart, which has been modi-

A Convincing Experiment

In 1949, anatomist James B. Hamilton, MD, performed landmark research into the causes of baldness in an experiment that predated the work of Dr. Orentreich by six years. Dr. Hamilton based his experiment on the observation that eunuchs—men who have been castrated, and, therefore, do not produce testosterone—maintain the hairline they had at the time of castration.

Working with a population of castrated convicts, Dr. Hamilton divided his subjects into two groups: those with a family history of baldness, and those without. He then began injecting the men in both groups with testosterone.

The men with a family history of baldness began to lose hair within weeks. Those without this history did not show signs of significant baldness. Interestingly, the hairlines of some men—those who were castrated prior to or during puberty—began to mature to an adult configuration. This led Dr. Hamilton to hypothesize that baldness, although triggered by the testosterone, was controlled by genetics. Time also seemed to be a factor, because the older the man, the faster his baldness progressed upon receiving the initial injections.

When Dr. Hamilton stopped the injections, he observed that the baldness immediately stopped progressing. This indicated that both testosterone and the proper genetic background were necessary to produce the expression of baldness.

fied for clarity. As you can see, in the early stages of male pattern baldness—Types I and II—some men begin to experience baldness in the temporal zones (the temple area), while others start losing the hair along the forehead (the frontal hairline). During these stages, the hair at the crown (vertex) and on the back of the head is beginning to thin as well, although this thinning is not obvious.

As the baldness progresses into Type III, in which the hair loss is considered mild, some men experience increased balding above the temples, while others find greater recessions in the forehead area, as seen in Type IIIa. Hair loss may also begin at the crown—Type III vertex—during this stage. Those whose hair loss has progressed to Type IV experience more extensive balding above the temples or, like Type IVa, will notice that their frontal hairlines are continuing to recede. In some men, the loss may also become more noticeable at the crown. Type V is considered significant in terms of hair loss. In most cases, the hair is lost from the top and crown areas of the head, and the fringe area is beginning to decrease. Hair loss is considered extensive for those in the Type VI category. Most of the head is bald, but the fringe area is about the same size as that in Type V. Those who reach Type VII (and not all men do) experience severe hair loss. At this point, the entire top of the head and crown is bald and the fringe area is markedly diminished.

Not all of the reasons for patterned hair-loss differences in men

THE LUDWIG CHART

This chart shows the typical progressive stages of female pattern baldness. Note the retention of the frontal hairline in each stage.

Ludwig Classification	Description
TYPE I 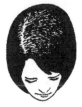	• Hair in the forelock area (behind the frontal hairline) is at the earliest stage of hair loss. ***Considered minimal thinning.***
TYPE II 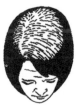	• In Type II, the thinning has progressed to a noticeable point. ***Considered moderate thinning.***
TYPE III 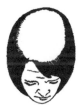	• In Type III, the thinning has progressed to a very noticeable degree. ***Considered extensive thinning.***

The Ludwig Chart (above) and the Norwood Classification Chart (pages 50–51) are reprinted with permission from: Olsen, EA. "Androgenetic alopecia" in: Disorders of Hair Growth: Diagnosis and Treatment. Olsen, EA (ed). New York: McGraw-Hill, 1994.

THE NORWOOD CLASSIFICATION CHART (Types I–III)

The following chart describes the common hair loss patterns that occur during male pattern baldness. The hair loss in Types I through III is considered minimal to moderate.

NORWOOD CLASSIFICATION	DESCRIPTION
Type I	• Hairline is at the earliest stage of hair loss with very minimal, if any, recession.
Type II	• Type II shows a slight recession of the frontal hairline, and more noticeable hair loss at the temples, which form definite "triangles."
Type IIa	• In Type IIa, the frontal hairline has receded and is high on the forehead. ***Considered minimal hair loss.***
Type III	• Type III is characterized by deep temple recessions.
Type IIIa	• In Type IIIa, the frontal hair loss is almost to the midpoint of the top of the head.
Type III (vertex)	• Loss may also begin at the crown, as seen in Type III (vertex). This is the first stage in which the hair loss is considered "baldness." ***Considered mild hair loss.***

THE NORWOOD CLASSIFICATION CHART (Types IV–VII)

The hair loss in Types IV through VII is more extensive, ranging from moderate to severe. As you can see, not all balding men fit precisely into a single defined class.

NORWOOD CLASSIFICATION	DESCRIPTION
Type IV	• Type IV has frontal and temporal hair loss that extends beyond that seen in Type III. A band of hair across the top of the head joins the fringes.
Type IVa	• In Type IVa, the hair loss extends beyond the midpoint of the top of the scalp. *Considered moderate hair loss.*
Type V	• In Type V, the band of hair on top of the head has thinned significantly.
Type Va	• Type Va has hair loss that extends to the crown area. *Considered significant hair loss.*
Type VI	• The band of hair on top of the head is now gone as the frontal baldness connects with the baldness at the crown. *Considered extensive hair loss.*
Type VII	• The only remaining hair is in a "horseshoe" band of fringe. *Considered severe hair loss.*

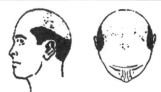

and women are completely understood; however, one obvious explanation is that women have less testosterone than men. They also have less DHT, which spares them from the same extensive hair loss that is often seen in men. As discussed earlier, testosterone is converted to DHT with the aid of the enzyme 5 alpha-reductase. Women have only half the amount of this enzyme as men, and they have even less in their scalp. What their scalps *do* have are significant levels of *aromatase,* an enzyme that is believed to block the formation of DHT. Aromatase is present in especially high concentrations in the frontal hairlines of most women, which may explain why their hairlines are resistant to balding.

Diffuse Alopecia

Diffuse alopecia is a subcategory of androgenetic alopecia. It has similar causes as male pattern baldness, but never progresses to complete baldness. There are three types of diffuse alopecia: unpatterned, patterned, and senile.

Diffuse unpatterned alopecia is characterized by a general thinning of the hair over the entire head (including the fringe area). In rare instances, the thinning occurs in random patches. This condition is much more common in women than it is in men.

Those with *diffuse patterned alopecia* have hair that thins noticeably in the same specific pattern that is seen in common male pattern baldness. The hair loss, however, never reaches full baldness. This type of alopecia can occur in both sexes; it is the most common type of androgenetic hair loss in women.

Senile alopecia refers to a general thinning of the hair as one ages. It is called "senile" because it tends to manifest as one reaches advanced age, usually after age sixty. Senile alopecia affects both men and women equally.

Alopecia Areata

Alopecia areata is characterized by complete baldness in random but clearly defined patches on the scalp. In this condition, which is considered an autoimmune disease, the individual's immune system actually attacks the hair follicles in the affected area. In severe cases, called *alopecia totalis,* the hair loss can involve the entire scalp and may include the eyebrows and eyelashes. And those with *alopecia universalis*—the most severe type—experience hair loss over the entire body. Currently, there is no known cure for alopecia areata, however there are treatments, including steroids, Retin-A, oral zinc, immuno-suppressive drugs, and ultraviolet light treatment. In some instances, this condition will spontaneously reverse itself.

Anagen Effluvium

Anagen effluvium is characterized by loss of hair in the anagen (growth) phase. Since approximately 90 percent of the hairs on one's head are in the anagen phase, this condition is associated with marked thinning over the entire scalp.

Typically, anagen effluvium is caused by anticancer drugs, x-ray therapy, or toxic drugs such as arsenic, bismuth, colchicine, borax, gold, and thallium. When the offending agent is discontinued, the hair loss will stop. Then the follicles will resume their normal activity, and hair will begin to grow again.

Telogen Effluvium

Telogen effluvium is characterized by an unusually large number of follicles entering a telogen (resting) phase, followed by hair loss in those follicles. The result is often significant and dramatic thinning. However, this type of hair loss is temporary, as the new anagen hairs will begin growing in place of those that were shed.

There are numerous causes of telogen effluvium, including hormonal changes associated with childbirth or termination of a pregnancy, illnesses associated with high fevers, or surgery of any type. Chronic conditions such as diabetes, thyroid conditions, anemia, or systemic lupus erythematosis are other possible causes. Stress caused by crash diets, severe mental anxiety, and various drugs or medications (see the inset on page 54) may induce this type of hair loss as well.

Finally, a localized telogen effluvium, more commonly known as *shock loss*, can result from hair transplant surgery. When incisions are made to receive hair grafts, the blood supply to the hair follicles in the surrounding area may be temporarily interrupted,

Pharmaceutical Causes of Telogen Effluvium

The drugs and medications listed below are considered possible causes of telogen effluvium. Product brand names are provided in parentheses.

Angiotensin-Converting Enzyme Inhibitors
captopril (Capoten)
enalapril (Vasotec)

Antacids
cimetidine (Tagamet)
famotidine (Pepcid)

Anticoagulants
heparin
warfarin (Coumadin)

Anticonvulsants
carbamazepine (Tegretol)
phenytoin (Dilantin)
valproate (Depakote)

Antithyroid Drugs
iodine
propylthiouracil (PTU)

Beta Blockers
acebutolol (Sectral)
atenolol (Tenormin)
labetalol (Trandate)
metoprolol (Lopressor)
nadolol (Corgard)
pindolol (Visken)
propranolol (Inderol)
timolol (Blocadren)

Calcium Channel Blockers
verapamil (Calan)
diltiazem (Cardizem)

Cholesterol Reduction
cholestyramine (Questran)
clofibrate (Atromid)

Retinoids
isotretinoin (Accutane)
Vitamin A overdose

resulting in some hair loss. However, the hair will begin to grow again within two or three months.

Self-Induced Hair Loss

There are two main types of self-induced hair loss—traction alopecia and trichotillomania. *Traction alopecia* is caused by prolonged physical tension on the hair, such as that caused by wearing very tight braids or corn rows. Over time, the hair is literally pulled out. Those who wear certain hair additions, such as extenders, are also at risk for traction alopecia because these additions are attached to existing hair. Over time, the constant pull against the follicles may cause hair loss. The area of hair under the most tension will experience the most significant baldness, leaving a shape or "pattern" that is specific to that area. Although some hair may grow back, traction alopecia tends to be a permanent condition.

Trichotillomania is a term coined by a French dermatologist in the late 1800s to describe the compulsion he saw in patients who continuously plucked out their hair. This psychological condition most commonly affects children, adolescents, and women. Typically, those with trichotillomania, pull out the hair from their scalp in distinct patches. Some pluck out their eyebrows and eyelashes, as well. Although this condition is manageable with counseling, the resulting hair loss can be permanent.

Scarring Alopecias

Scarring alopecias, which are the result of destroyed hair follicles, are characterized by patchy hair loss in discreet areas of the scalp. There are many causes for this type of loss, including inherited abnormalities of the skin and hair follicles; bacterial, fungal, or viral infections; and tumors of the skin. Disorders such as lupus, lichen planus, pseudopelade of Brocq, and Sjögren's syndrome, as well as illnesses or conditions like syphilis and scleroderma, may cause scarring alopecias as well.

For those with these disorders, treating the hair loss is secondary to caring for the condition that is causing it. Examination and treatment by a physician is important.

MORE ABOUT HAIR LOSS IN WOMEN

Although we have already discussed the causes of hair loss in women, a few additional points merit attention. Women represent 40 percent of the total population in the United States experiencing hair loss—more than most people realize. And by age sixty, approximately 50 percent of all women lose their hair to some degree. Unlike men, the manifestation of hair loss in women is usually very gradual, with the rate accelerating at menopause. Losing hair also tends to be more easily affected by hormonal changes, medical conditions, and stress, although this type of loss is usually temporary.

The management of women with hair loss is quite different than it is for men, requiring significant expertise in both the diagnosis and treatment. As you will see in the following chapters, women for whom surgical hair rearrangement is indicated require special surgical skills to achieve the best results.

CONCLUSION

So there you have it—the truth about what causes baldness and what doesn't. This awareness will help you accurately assess the various surgical and nonsurgical treatments that are available today. The chapters in Part II present these options.

PART II

The Options

4

Cosmetic Hair Additions

"There's no time for a man to recover his hair that grows bald by nature."

—WILLIAM SHAKESPEARE, *COMEDY OF ERRORS*

osmetic hair additions are a great means of restoring the appearance of a full head of hair. Today's improved materials and techniques result in additions that can appear quite natural, both in color and texture. In addition, this type of hair replacement often allows for participation in the most vigorous of sports and other physical activities. In order to choose the type of cosmetic hair addition that is right for you, it's important to understand all of the options.

This chapter presents all of the aspects of hair additions, including their components, designs, and cost. It explains the various attachment methods, and shows how additions can be an effective solution—either temporary or permanent—for hair loss.

WHAT IS A HAIR ADDITION?

What were known for years as hairpieces, transformations, or toupees, are now more commonly called hair replacements, hair additions, or hair systems. These include commercially advertised products such as extensions, weaves, integrations, fusions, and nonsurgical grafts. They supply hair quickly, efficiently, and affordably. Furthermore, anyone, no matter what age, can safely wear this type of hair addition if it is properly fitted.

COMPONENTS OF A HAIR ADDITION

Virtually every hair addition is made up of the same basic components: the base, the hair (synthetic or real), and a method of attachment. Over the years, companies have combined these components in different ways to achieve a wide variety of hair additions—something to satisfy everyone, regardless of concerns about price, appearance, ease of use, and/or maintenance.

The Base

The base is the main structural component of a hair addition, giving it shape and contour. Modern synthetic materials, particularly polyurethane and nylon, have substantially improved the quality of bases. These man-made fibers repel body oils and moisture, are durable, and retain their shape even after prolonged use.

Most bases are designed with several factors in mind. As the foundation for a hair addition, the base must serve as an anchor that provides a stable surface for attachment to the scalp or existing hair. Because it lies directly against the head, the base should also be as smooth and comfortable as possible. Most important, it should be ultra-thin to minimize the possibility of detection, especially during close inspection. If someone runs a hand through your hair, you don't want the base to feel like a foreign object.

The material used for the base also determines the way in which the fibers (hairs) are attached to it. For example, a polyester or nylon mesh base requires the added hair fibers to be knotted to it, while polyurethane and silicone bases allow the fibers to be either knotted *or* looped. Knotting and looping each have trade offs—durability versus appearance. The knotting process creates a small visible "speck" at the base of the hair that may allow for some detectability. The looping process, although less likely to be detected, may result in fibers that are less durable and more easily lost.

One of the biggest drawbacks of hair additions is their difficulty in creating a natural-looking frontal hairline. Generally, the fronts of most additions are simply extensions of the base. Because a base needs to be strong and durable, it often cannot be thin enough to realistically create the look of a typical male frontal hairline. In addition, matching the skin color in this very visible area is difficult, especially for those who desire to comb their hair back or away from the forehead.

There have been several attempts toward eliminating this frontal hairline problem. For example, new skin-like bases made of silicone or polyurethane are micro-thin, and scalloped along the base's edge for better blending with the skin. Other fine mesh bases are made of polyester or nylon. All are colored to match the skin. The fronts that are made of these materials tend to be fairly durable. The thicker the material, the more durable the front—and the more noticeable.

Another way some manufactureres deal with the frontal hairline problem is by adding hair to an extra-fine "lace-type" front, which blends naturally into the skin at the hairline. This is an almost-forgotten method used on hairpieces worn by such classic screen legends as Humphrey Bogart, Bing Crosby, and Jimmy Stewart. Using current attachment methods with old-world lace fronts has dramatically changed the cosmetic hair business, significantly increasing styling options. It allows men to comb their hair straight back, up, or leave it "unstyled."

Initially, lace-type fronts were made of silk and cotton. They were extremely delicate and began to degrade after only a few months. And this problem only increased when they were coupled with additions that used permanent attachment methods. Today, well-crafted lace fronts are made of polyester and nylon, giving them a much longer life. Programs for lace-based systems usually include a monthly payment that covers replacement of the lace fronts or the entire addition as often as every two to three months when worn permanently. If it's your desire to wear your hair straight back and you can afford such a natural-looking addition, do it! However, if you are concerned with cost and maintenance, it might be wiser to consider a hairstyle that will cover the frontal hairline.

In addition to the actual material used, three other factors—length, curl, and color—can make the frontal hairline appear natural. A regular hair addition can be cut extremely short to fall forward in what some call a short Caesar cut. This style covers the hairline very well, and doesn't get messed up in the wind or during physical activity. Curl is another factor that can provide a more natural look to a base. To help camouflage a base's harshness, a small amount of "baby hair"—slightly frizzy or curly hair—is built into the first millimeter of the front. A scalloped front further softens the edge, giving it a more natural look. The third element required for a natural-looking addition is color. Making the first few rows of hair a lighter color than the rest helps them blend better with skin coloring.

The Hair

One common misconception about hair systems is that they are made with animal hair. Human hair makes up the vast majority of all additions, although very small amounts of yak or angora may be used to simulate white or gray hair. But even this limited role for animal hair is being discontinued and replaced by improved synthetic fibers, which offer realistic texture and color. Although human hair can create a slightly more natural appearance than synthetic, its color degrades faster. Exposure to the sun can cause human hair to fade after a month, while synthetic fibers retain their color for six to eight months. Human hair, however, can be recolored; synthetic types must be replaced.

India is the largest source of human hair for additions. Typically, this hair is medium in texture and can be used in most additions. Asia is another source, but provides only hair that is coarse, straight, and dark, which means its use is limited. Characteristically, the hair from western and northern Europe is fine textured and comes in various colors.

Modern synthetic hair fibers have improved greatly over the last decade. They repel body oil, are extremely durable, and retain their shape for a long time. Cyberhair, which is made of nylon, is an example of the new breed of synthetic fibers found in quality hair additions. This fiber, which reduces the need for maintenance and is easier to style, is changing the nature of the hair-addition business for the better. We'll be presenting more about Cyberhair later in this chapter.

Attachment Methods

For many years, the biggest problem with hair additions, even before the consideration of texture and color, has been the attachment method. Many additions come off easily, especially in the wind and during periods of physical activity. In 1995, a hair addition was put to the test during a boxing match between John-John Molina and Oscar de la Hoya. Molina wore an addition that remained perfectly in place during all twelve rounds of the bout, even after being drenched in sweat and pounded by de la Hoya. It was a testament to the technique of perimeter bonding (discussed on pages 65 and 66).

The two major attachment classifications—skin and hair—offer a variety of safe and effective options. Within each category, the attachments are further distinguished as either removable (taken off each day) or permanent (taken off every two to six weeks, depending on the system). In general, we tend to favor removable methods, whether attached to the skin or hair, for three reasons. First, cleaning the addition and the scalp is much easier. Second, some permanent attachments (hair weaving, knotting/fusion) can result in hair loss due to traction alopecia. Finally, there is the matter of cost. Typically, permanent additions need to be replaced about every ten months, while removable systems usually last twice as long.

Regular maintenance for most permanently attached hair additions takes about forty-five minutes to an hour. With removable additions, only the time required for a haircut may be necessary. If other services are needed, such as coloring and replacing lost hairs, the process may take longer. A professional should perform all permanent bonding applications and service on the additions. As for the removable types, a reliable retailer should take the time to give you clear instructions on proper application and removal methods.

Skin-Attachment Methods

There are several methods for attaching hair additions to the bald or balding scalp. Most of these methods fall into two categories—*adhesive* and *surgical*. A third category, *vacuum* or *suction*, does not require glue or surgery, and is most commonly used by those who have alopecia totalis or alopecia universalis (discussed in Chapter 3). To use a hairpiece with this type of attachment, the entire scalp must be either shaved bare or naturally bald. The suction created by the close fit of the base against the user's scalp keeps the hairpiece in place. Although this is not the most secure attachment method, it is extremely easy to use and much cleaner than using adhesives.

ADHESIVES

Tape and glues, called *sealants,* are the two most common types of adhesives used to attach a hair addition to the bare scalp. Both types can be quite secure.

Double-sided tape is the easiest sealant to use. It is usually placed on the addition, which is then positioned on the scalp. Depending on the individual's hair-loss pattern and bald areas, this placement will vary. Active individuals may choose to use tape around the entire perimeter of the addition for added security, while those with more sedentary lifestyles may use only a very small amount. Although it is easy to use, double-sided tape can sometimes leave undesirable residue on the scalp that may be difficult to remove. This isn't a problem if the tape is changed daily. Otherwise, a slow meltdown of the adhesive will occur, leaving a sticky residue. When using tape, the addition should be removed before bathing and while sleeping at night.

Waterproof glues can be used with removable hair systems for added security, especially during activities such as swimming. These sealants, which come in tubes or bottles, are applied directly to the two-sided tape. However, they should be removed every twenty-four to forty-eight hours with the appropriate solvent. The most effective sealants are made of either polymer resins or latex adhesives. Both are flexible, durable, easy to use and remove, and generally safe for skin contact.

For the technique called *full-head bonding,* which is considered a "nonsurgical" graft, the entire base is attached with an adhesive that lasts longer than the type used in removable additions. Many people like the security provided by this method. It also lasts about two weeks.

Possible allergic reaction is the most important consideration when using any type of sealant. Always test the product on a small area of skin before using it on your scalp. Also, be aware that retailers should have a manufacturer's Material Safety Data Sheet (MSDS) on the sealants they recommend. This sheet contains information on any known health risks associated with the products. Ask to see a copy. Also, ask the retailer if the company carries product liability coverage. This is the only way to insure the safety of your attachment. If the business cannot furnish you with the MSDS or proof of insurance, go elsewhere.

SURGICAL METHODS

Suturing and maxillofacial implants are the primary surgical attachment methods for hair additions. Due to the complexity of these processes and the potential for post-surgical problems, they must always be performed by a qualified doctor.

- **Suturing.** This permanent attachment technique involves sewing the addition directly to the scalp. It is a dangerous practice that invariably leads to infection and/or permanent scarring. Most individuals who bear scars from this procedure find themselves forced to wear hairpieces constantly to keep the scars covered.

- **Maxillofacial implants.** These implants are literally "snaps" that are surgically implanted in the skull and serve as anchors for the hair addition, which then snaps on. This method requires a firm and long-term commitment to wearing a hair addition, since one part of the snap attachment remains in the scalp. In addition, the expense of the snap mechanisms and the surgery to implant them is prohibitive. However, the chief concern with this method is its high infection rate, which can lead to osteomyelitis—a dangerous and painful bone infection.

Hair-Attachment Methods

As their name implies, the various hair-attachment methods use a person's remaining fringe hair as an anchor for the hairpiece. Because they offer security and durability during strenuous activity, these methods represent some of the most popular options used today. Most are permanent attachments.

- **Perimeter Bonding.** Today's most popular permanent hair-attachment method is perimeter bonding. It involves using an adhesive to bind the base of the hair addition directly to existing fringe hair, which has been shaved to a length of ⅛ inch. When done by a qualified professional, bonding is highly effective and wears well. Depending on how fast the fringe hair grows, the addition will remain affixed for a number of weeks. As the real hair grows, the addition will become loose. At this point, the hair is cut and the adhesive is removed from the addition. Then the bonding process is repeated. Remember to test for possible allergic reactions to the adhesive.

- **Weaving.** This attachment method involves tightly braiding existing hair around the perimeter of the balding area. The hair addition is then sewn to the braids, which serve as an anchor. The length of time between braiding sessions is usually between three to four weeks, depending on how fast the person's hair grows. While attached, the addition is washed right along with the hair, and any additional maintenance can be performed during its rebraiding. The downside of the weave is that the tight braiding can lead to traction alopecia.

- **Knotting/Fusion.** For this method of attachment, existing hair is pulled through eyelets at the edge of the hair addition's base and then knotted. For those with finely textured hair, sometimes an acrylic adhesive, such as butylcyanoacrylate or cyanoacrylate, is used to seal the knot, ensuring that it will stay. When an adhesive is used, the process is called *fusion*. Fusion is not a popular method because of the risk of traction alopecia.

- **Beading.** This attachment method is similar to knotting. Existing hair is pulled through eyelets at the edge of a hair addition's base, and then secured by small metal beads. Because of their size and location, these beads are barely visible to the casual observer. Just as in other attachment methods that rely on existing hair, traction alopecia is a concern.

- **Clipping.** For this easy-to-use attachment method, small clips of various sizes are attached to the underside of the hair addition. The addition is then clipped onto the existing hair and snapped closed for security. Although the hairpiece can be easily removed with this type of attachment, the clips can cause traction alopecia.

- **Micro Point Linking.** Micro Point Linking is a patented process that represents the first method of adding hair without adhesives, weaves, clips, or surgery. Effective for men and women with thinning hair, this process permanently links *Cyberhair*—a revolutionary synthetic fiber that looks and feels real—to existing hair. By knotting two pieces of Cyberhair (yielding four separate ends) to one existing hair, the density of that hair is increased by 400 percent. The process is completely safe and doesn't limit physical activities.

Arguably the most attractive technique available, Micro Point Linking is an option only for men and women who are in the early stages of hair loss. There must be enough real hair to serve as the base for the linked hair. Caring for the added hair is no different from caring for your own.

Micro Point Linking is labor intensive, often taking two or more hours per session during the initial process. And due to the natural shedding of hair, regular maintenance—usually every three to four weeks—is necessary. It is also a costly procedure, but many believe the results are worth it.

IS A HAIR ADDITION RIGHT FOR YOU?

Many individuals are excellent candidates for hair additions. And most men who wear them for a year will continue wearing them for the rest of their lives. This is especially true for those who choose the removable types. Those who wear permanent additions tend to have higher cancellation rates because of the trips they are required to make to the stylist every four to six weeks for proper maintenance.

What do hair additions offer that the other options—surgery and pharmaceuticals—don't? Two advantages are obvious. First, the change in appearance is immediate. You don't have to wait eight months after surgery or take pills for six months before seeing changes. From the moment you put on the hair addition, your appearance is altered. Second, the health risks involved are minimal. Attachment methods can pose the only potential problems, and most have no harmful side effects at all.

Another advantage of hair additions is that most come with

money back guarantees, usually within thirty days. You certainly can't get that kind of assurance with surgery. With removable additions, you also have a great deal of flexibility in choosing when to wear them. Pharmaceutical options, for example, require daily compliance, and results are not guaranteed, even when directions are followed. Finally, hair additions can provide more coverage and density than the other options.

There are two types of men for whom hair additions are an especially good option. The first type includes those who are balding at a very young age, particularly in their teens. For a seventeen-year-old male, a hair addition is the best short-term answer because it can immediately make him look normal, as compared to his contemporaries. Besides, surgery is never appropriate for anyone so young. By the time he's out of college, that young man can rethink all of his options, and decide what he wants to do in the long run. The second type of men for whom hair additions are a good option are those who cannot accept the inherent restrictions of surgery, such as limited coverage or less than "full" density. For these men, a hair addition is the perfect alternative. It provides coverage without permanent consequences.

Many women are excellent candidates for hair additions because they are likely to be more familiar and comfortable with wigs. Some have already worn them for fun or to temporarily alter their appearance. Because of the nature of female baldness, which was explained in Chapter 3, hair additions are often the best option, both as short- and long-term solutions for hair loss.

HOW TO BUY A HAIR ADDITION

Buying a hair addition is a major decision that should be approached with care and concern. However, try not to be too serious during the process. Keep in mind that you are doing something good for yourself. You are taking action to improve your appearance in a way that will bring you satisfaction. Maintain a positive attitude.

Find a Good Hair-Addition Provider

Finding a qualified provider is more than half the battle in getting a good product. This specialist must possess a number of important qualities, including the following:

- **Experience.** A qualified provider must have the skill to match a hair addition with the color and texture of your natural hair growth. He or she must be able to determine which hairstyle best complements your head and face. In other words, the provider should be experienced.

- **Compassion.** The person who sells you a hair addition should also be a good listener. He or she should be willing to talk (and listen) to you, understand what you want, and know how to best meet your needs. You are making a major decision about your appearance and shouldn't feel as if you are in this alone.

- **Integrity.** Professional integrity is critical in a hair provider. He or she must stand behind the work and do whatever is necessary to satisfy you as the client. Such integrity comes from experience and commitment to service.

You will be able to determine if your hair-addition provider has these qualities by talking to him or her and by checking references. Ask to have a number of past and current clients get in touch with you. Then set up meetings to discuss their experiences with the hair system and the company, and to see for yourself how the actual addition looks. Never ask for a client's number to make the call yourself. It is unethical and unprofessional for a company to disperse such information. We also recommend that clients meet privately, because most people tend to be more open and honest in such an atmosphere.

Another possible consideration is company background. How long has it been in existence? Does it appear to be a company that will be around ten, fifteen, twenty years from now? Keep in mind that you may choose a hair system that requires regular maintenance over the long haul.

Choose an Addition That Best Fits Your Needs

Once you have chosen your provider, you'll be able to work toward getting a hair addition that will best meet your needs. Although everyone has different requirements, depending on lifestyle, budget, existing hair color, and so on, there are certain general guidelines that can help ensure product satisfaction.

First, make sure the person who is going to design or style your hair addition knows exactly what you want. For this, we strongly urge you to bring photographs of the look you hope to achieve. We can't stress enough how important this is. The designer must have a clear understanding of what you want—the pictures should be focused, and the desired hairstyle easy to see. Sometimes it is helpful to bring in photos of a younger you with hair, so the designer can see how you once looked. This will aid in creating a hairpiece that appears more natural. Photographs, however, are good only for initial design concerns. Viewing yourself with the actual addition is the only way to accurately assess how natural it will look.

Don't become a "do-it-yourself" expert and restrict the designer in any aspect of the addition from the type of materials used to the amount of hair to be included. Once you have found a good company and feel confident with it, let the experts do their job. If you have been clear as to what you want, they should be able to design a quality hairpiece to your liking. Remember that fittings and small adjustments will be necessary to get it just right, and don't be disappointed or angry if it takes several. The company is only trying to satisfy you.

A good company should offer guaranteed satisfaction for its products. Never sign a contract guaranteeing payment for a hair addition before you actually see yourself in it—unless, of course, it specifically allows for a *full* refund. Some companies offer refunds but may also require a small nonrefundable deposit for processing the order. Just be sure that this is stated in the contract.

All hair additions require maintenance, and anyone who says differently is either lying or uninformed. After getting an addition, make sure the company provides you with all the necessary items to maintain it, including a schedule for "tune-ups." In addition to proper care, other factors have a direct impact on the longevity of the product. For instance, is your system attached permanently? Is the system made of lace? An average good-quality system can be worn for up to eighteen months if it is removed daily; but that same unit may wear out in three months to a year if worn permanently. Lace fronts and very thin polyurethane bases will wear out two to three times faster than those made of more durable material.

We also recommend finding a good hair-addition provider that is within fifty miles of either your home or workplace. Close proximity will make it easier for you to return for regularly scheduled service appointments and other matters.

If you do your homework—properly research the available options and find a qualified provider—you can succeed in getting a hair addition that fulfills your needs. Of course, if one can succeed, one can also fail. Failure means getting something that looks unnatural or detectable. Usually, this happens because the addition is inappropriate for the wearer's age—it is too dense, too dark in color, or just too big. Is it any wonder that people joke about hair additions, calling them rugs, hair helmets, and dead animal pelts? The typical sixty-year-old man doesn't have a hairline that touches his eyebrows. Nor does he have jet-black hair that is thicker than deep shag carpeting. A well-designed hair addition should be virtually undetectable to the casual observer. See the photos on page 72 for some examples.

COSTS OF HAIR ADDITIONS

Depending on their type and quality, hair-addition packages can range anywhere from $300 to upwards of $20,000. With so many options available, as an educated consumer, it's important to have an idea of the various costs involved.

For a removable hair addition, the average annual cost is between $1,200 and $2,400. This includes the price of the addition, regularly scheduled servicing, haircuts, and repairs. For a permanent system, the average annual cost ranges from $1,600 to $3,200. Prices for the Micro Point Link process will vary according to the number of strands used—typically, this means from $50 to $300 about every four weeks. For weaving, bonding, and fusion, the average price, which may include a haircut, is about $35 to $50 every four to six weeks. A vacuum-fitted prosthesis usually runs anywhere from $2,500 and up.

Some people fool themselves into believing that hair additions are cheaper alternatives to surgery, but this is not necessarily so.

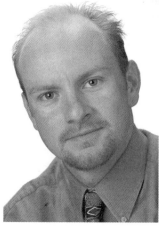
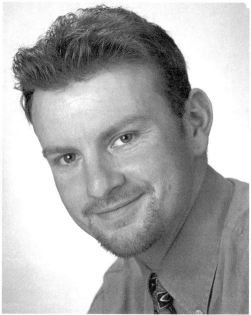
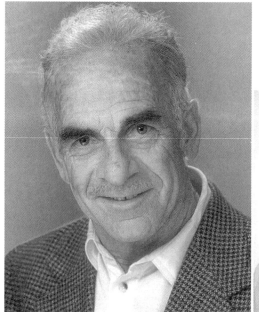
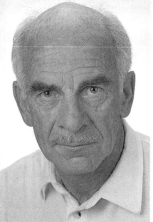

Photographs courtesy of Mike Mahoney of iwanthair.com.

WELL-DESIGNED HAIR ADDITIONS

Attention to the right color and texture, as well as proper size and fit,
is what characterizes a natural-looking, undetectable hair addition.

It is important to be aware of this during the decision-making process. A colleague of ours who works in a well-known facility told us that his company expects an income of about $12,600 over a five-year period for each hair system sold. This reflects the cost of two hair additions (the original and one replacement), monthly maintenance, and repairs. So you see, maintaining a hair system can be more expensive during the first five years of use than a permanent surgical solution.

SOME FINAL CONSIDERATIONS

There's another interesting point to consider before choosing a hair addition. Once a person wears one, he can become "addicted" to having lots of hair, which can make "weaning" difficult. Many clients who have worn hair systems for many years have reported that as they get older, they would be satisfied being bald or having thin hair. However, because they have worn hairpieces for so long, they believe the change would be too dramatic, so they reluctantly continue wearing them.

Finally, when you decide to try a hair system, be sure that the seller doesn't shave your head (even partially) until you have committed to the system. When using an addition that requires shaved areas of the head, it's important to realize that if you elect to stop wearing it, you may have to shave your head entirely. Otherwise, you will have isolated bald spots.

CONCLUSION

Cosmetic hair additions are a good solid hair-replacement option for many. Recent advances, such as durable synthetic fibers with natural texture and color, have helped make additions less obvious. And such technology continues to improve.

Now that you have basic knowledge of hair additions, it's time to move on to Chapter 5, where the best pharmaceutical options available in the field of hair replacement will be presented.

5.

Pharmaceutical Options

It's nearly impossible to flip through a magazine, watch television, or navigate the Internet without hearing about some product that claims to prevent, reverse, or cure baldness. With such an abundance of so-called "miracle" products vying for attention, it has become increasingly difficult to identify the legitimate merchandise from the snake oil. That is, of course, unless you do your homework.

This chapter presents current pharmaceutical options—pills, lotions, and shampoos—that can potentially stimulate hair growth. Many of these remedies work well alone or in conjunction with cosmetic hair additions or surgery. Depending on your personal goals, some of these options may be excellent solutions for you. But one thing is important to understand from the beginning—at this time, there are no pharmaceuticals that can "cure" baldness. There is nothing out there that can reverse or completely prevent hair loss.

THE PRODUCTS

Of the many products available on the market today, we will be presenting the ones that merit attention in the treatment of male pattern baldness (androgenetic alopecia). These include the FDA-approved pharmaceuticals minoxidil and finasteride, as well as dutasteride—a drug recently developed for the treatment of enlarged prostate. We'll also discuss ketoconazole, a medication that has been shown to have positive effects in treating hair loss. In addition to these legitimate remedies, we'll talk about a number of "natural" treatments that have become popular, but whose effectiveness is suspect.

Other than minoxidil, finasteride, dutasteride, and ketoconazole, no other drugs or treatments, including the "laser" comb, have been proven through scientific testing to reverse, slow, or stop hair loss. Without scientifically controlled studies, there is no way to qualify or quantify a product's expected results, nor is there any way to estimate an individual's chance at success with it.

Minoxidil

Rogaine was first introduced in the United States in 1988, and was the first prescription medication expressly used to treat male pattern baldness. Its active ingredient, minoxidil, was developed by Upjohn Pharmaceuticals (now owned by Pfizer), and is the same ingredient in Loniten, a drug taken orally to lower blood pressure. Minoxidil's effectiveness in hair growth was discovered accidentally when some patients who were taking the medication to lower their blood pressure experienced hair growth all over their bodies, a condition called *hypertrichosis*. Minoxidil, however, could not be prescribed as an oral medication to treat hair loss because of its effect on blood pressure. As a result, Upjohn researchers developed Rogaine—a topically applied formulation containing minoxidil.

Minoxidil was available as a 2% concentration for many years exclusively from Upjohn, who held the patent. In 1996, when the company's patent ended, a number of drug companies began selling "minoxidil 2%." Upjohn responded by conducting clinical trials of a 5% minoxidil solution, now available as Rogaine extra-strength. Upjohn holds the patent on this particular solution; however, other companies can offer 5% solutions as well. The products sold in a generic form often contain additional ingredients, such as Retin-A, steroids, zinc, and grape seed extract, to distinguish them from Upjohn's and, presumably, to enhance the results. Minoxidil is the only scientifically tested and approved over-the-counter treatment.

How It Works

Through scalp biopsies, scientists have observed that minoxidil enlarges and revitalizes shrunken intermediate hair follicles, stimulating them to grow terminal hairs again (see Understanding Intermediate Hair Follicles below). Minoxidil cannot, however, grow new hairs from dead follicles. To act, the solution must be rubbed directly on the scalp, not on the hair itself, twice a day. Somewhat messy to handle, this product's oily texture often leaves the hair sticky and difficult to style.

Effectiveness

Extensive trials were performed on Rogaine. The original study examined 126 men with Norwood Type III to Type VI patterns (see pages 50 and 51), who had experienced hair loss for anywhere from two to thirty years. The subjects ranged in age from twenty to forty years old. The twelve-month study evaluated treatment with 2% and 3% topical minoxidil and a placebo. The results showed no statistical difference between the two strengths of minoxidil; however, there was a difference when compared to the placebo.

The hair counts showed that the medication caused an average of 218 new terminal hairs to grow in a one-inch-diameter circle over the baseline number of hairs. A follow-up study, examining the effectiveness of continued use after five years, showed that on average there was a gradual decline in terminal hair counts from the maximum achieved at one year, but this number didn't fall

---

Understanding Intermediate Hair Follicles

Intermediate hair follicles are those in the "intermediate" stage between a normal active follicle and one that is dead. Smaller in size than anagen follicles that produce terminal hairs, intermediate follicles produce hair that is thinner and lighter in color. Over time, the follicles continue to shrink until they produce only tiny vellus hairs, commonly known as "peach fuzz." The active ingredients in products like Rogaine and Propecia either stimulate intermediate hair follicles to regrow terminal hairs or slow the miniaturization of terminal follicles.

below the initial baseline count. According to the study, at the four-and-a-half- to five-year mark, the average number of hairs above baseline in this group of men (a different group from the initial study) was 211 in a one-inch-diameter circle, compared to 273 above baseline at one year.

During clinical trials for its 5% minoxidil solution, Upjohn assessed the difference in hair growth between Rogaine 2% and 5% solutions. After forty-eight weeks, the 5% solution resulted in the growth of 95 hairs in a one-inch-diameter circle over the baseline number. Those who used the 2% solution showed growth of 65 hairs, while the subjects in the placebo group experienced growth of 20 hairs. Using a subjective evaluation, researchers also concluded that the 5% solution provided nearly three times greater improvement in scalp coverage than the 2% solution.

To enhance minoxidil's absorption, some physicians recommend using Retin-A along with it. Although Retin-A may, in fact, increase minoxidil's absorption, it does not necessarily increase hair growth. Furthermore, it can cause scalp irritation and increased sensitivity to the sun. Upjohn has stated (and we agree) that Rogaine (and other hair products containing minoxidil) should not be used with any agents, including Retin-A. Those who elect to use this combination should do so with great caution and only while under the watchful eye of a physician.

The Risks

Minoxidil's potential side effects include scalp irritation, redness, itching, and scaling, but such symptoms occur in less than 10 out of every 100 users. For some, these problems can become serious enough to force the discontinuation of the therapy; however, they are not permanent and will resolve once the treatment is stopped. In very rare instances, minoxidil may enter the bloodstream, causing symptoms such as headache, blurred vision, irregular heartbeat, lightheadedness, and tingling or swelling of the hands and feet. In some instances, women who use minoxidil experience excess hair growth in areas where the product was not applied—usually the face and arms. Once the treatment is discontinued, this side effect reverses itself.

Although the heart medication Loniten also contains minoxidil as its active ingredient, it should never be taken for the treatment of hair loss. Its potential to cause significant and dangerous drops in blood pressure can lead to fainting and even stroke. However, if you have both hair loss *and* high blood pressure, you may want to speak to your doctor about this product. Just keep in mind that Loniten stimulates hair growth over the entire body, not just the head.

Rogaine for Women

In the initial clinical study by Upjohn examining the effects of Rogaine's 2% formula on women aged eighteen to forty-five, 40 percent of the subjects experienced minimal hair growth after eight months, while 19 percent showed moderate growth.

Although formal studies have not been performed on women using a 5% minoxidil solution, it has been our experience that it is more effective in stimulating hair growth on women than the 2% solution. Because minoxidil is excreted in breast milk, neither formulation is recommended for women who are breastfeeding. Of course, we also make our interested female clients aware of the other possible side effects of the medication, such as scalp irritation and facial hair growth. If the latter side effect is noted while taking the 5% minoxidil solution, a switch to the 2% solution is recommended.

Finasteride

Released as a prescription medication in 1998, Propecia is the first medication created to specifically address the biochemical cause of hair loss as it is understood at this time. Its active ingredient is finasteride, which was developed by Merck & Co. Finasteride is the same ingredient found in Proscar, a drug introduced in 1992 to combat *benign prostatic hyperplasia (BPH)*—enlargement of the prostate gland. Propecia tablets contain 1 milligram of finasteride, while Proscar contains 5 milligrams.

How It Works

In Chapter 3, you learned that testosterone is converted to dihydrotestosterone (DHT) by the enzyme 5 alpha-reductase ($5\alpha R$), and it is the presence of DHT that triggers baldness. Finasteride works by inhibiting or "blocking" the 5αR enzyme from forming DHT. Scalp biopsies have indicated that finasteride treatment results in lowered levels of DHT in the scalp tissue, which means, of course, that less DHT is interacting with the hair follicles. The decreased DHT levels allow some intermediate follicles to enlarge and regrow normal terminal hairs. Unlike Rogaine or other minoxidil products, which are applied topically, Propecia is taken orally.

Effectiveness

The Propecia studies included 1,879 men between the ages of eighteen and forty-one who were experiencing minimal to moderate hair loss in the anterior mid-scalp (top) or vertex (back) areas (see Figure 5.1 below). Prone to hair loss, these areas were of particular interest to researchers.

The study results were impressive. For the subjects who had been experiencing hair loss in the *vertex area,* the study revealed that after twenty-four months, 83 percent of the men taking Propecia grew visible terminal hairs while only 17 percent lost hair. Of the men who took the placebo, 72 percent continued losing their hair. At the end of the first year, the actual hair counts showed that those in the treated group gained an average of 86 hairs in the one-inch-diameter test circle. Those taking the placebo lost an average of 21 hairs in the test area. From this data, it was determined that, on average, men taking Propecia had approximately 107 more hairs in the test area than those not taking the medication.

Photographic assessment by a panel of dermatologists, who did not know which subjects were taking Propecia and which were

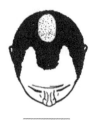

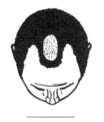

FIGURE 5.1. AREAS ASSESSED DURING PROPECIA STUDIES

Vertex
(back or crown)

Anterior Mid-scalp
(top)

on the placebo, evaluated the subjects after two years. Of those taking Propecia, 5 percent showed great improvement, 31 percent showed moderate improvement, 30 percent showed slight improvement, and 33 percent showed no further visible hair loss from the baseline assessment. Of the placebo group, only 7 percent experienced a slight improvement. The remainder of this group showed either some hair loss or no change.

For the subjects who had been experiencing hair loss in the *anterior mid-scalp area,* those taking Propecia had about 60 more hairs in the one-inch-diameter test circle than those in the placebo group. (Comparatively, those in the vertex study had 107 more hairs than the group taking the placebo.) The photographic assessment revealed that 4 percent in the treatment group showed moderate improvement, 34 percent had slight improvement, and 62 percent showed no additional loss. The placebo group had only 7 percent of the subjects showing slight improvement, while 85 percent had no apparent loss. The remaining 7 percent experienced visible hair loss.

Interestingly, in the studies involving the vertex area of the scalp, the men's hair continued to thicken visibly after the first year, although there was no increase in the number of terminal hairs. This is explained by Propecia's ability to increase hair shaft diameter, a factor that has a great effect on hair volume or hair mass—more so than an increased number of hairs. You see, by doubling the number of hairs, you are simply doubling the hair volume. But when doubling the diameter of the hair shaft, the hair volume is quadrupled, even though there is no change in the actual number of hairs.

Part of the initial two-year study was designed to answer the question, "What happens if I stop taking Propecia?" So some men took the treatment for the first year, and the placebo for the second. During the second year while on the placebo, these subjects lost the hair they had gained during the first year and returned to their pretreatment stage within twelve months.

A follow-up study, examining the effectiveness of the continued use of Propecia after the initial two years, was also performed. Individuals taking Propecia for five years when compared to those taking the placebo showed more hair in the vertex area—an average of 277 more hairs in a one-inch-diameter test circle. At the end of the fifth year, 65 percent of the subjects taking the treatment maintained or improved their hair count as compared to the count at the beginning of the study, while all of those receiving a placebo for five years lost hair. The photographic assessment done at the end of the five-year study rated 90 percent of the men who were taking the medication as either showing improvement or having no further visible hair loss from the initial baseline evaluation. Only 25 percent of the men taking the placebo had the same results.

Based on the information from these studies, Propecia can help treat hair loss in several ways. First, it can halt or slow down the hair-loss process; second, it can increase the number of cosmetically significant terminal hairs; and finally, it can take a population of intermediate hairs and increase shaft diameter, which builds hair volume.

To date, no studies on the effectiveness of using a combination of both Rogaine (or another minoxidil product) and Propecia have been conducted on humans. However, one study using stumptail macaque monkeys as subjects suggests that using a combination of both treatments is more effective than using either one alone. As both products are safe, you may choose to try them separately or in combination to see which works best.

Even with the varied and often modest hair-growth results for certain parts of the head, finasteride is an excellent enzyme blocker that can significantly decrease DHT levels. Some researchers believe there may be a reason Propecia doesn't get better results than it does. Propecia's active ingredient—finasteride—blocks only the Type II 5 α-reductase enzyme, which contributes about two-thirds of the DHT in the blood. However, it does not block the Type I 5 α-reductase enzyme, which produces the remaining third of DHT. It is for this reason that many researchers feel Propecia's ability to stimulate hair growth is limited.

Risks for Men

During the studies, Propecia's side effects were limited to decreased libido (diminished interest in sex), erectile dysfunction, and ejaculation disorder (mostly a decrease in semen, but not a decrease in sperm). It's important to note that only a very small percentage of the study subjects experienced these effects. Of those who were taking Propecia, 1.8 percent experienced a decrease in libido compared with 1.3 percent of those taking the placebo. Erectile dysfunction was seen in 1.3 percent of the men taking the medication, compared with 0.7 percent of those on the placebo. Finally, 1.2 percent experienced an ejaculation disorder, compared with 0.7 percent of those taking the placebo.

Although statistically, these differences are not significant, some men taking Propecia might notice slight signs or changes in these areas. What's important to keep in mind is that these side effects are completely reversible within a few days once the treatment is stopped. Furthermore, 58 percent of men who experienced these sexual changes yet continued taking the drug, also noticed that the changes were resolved within several weeks.

The use of finasteride, as either Proscar or Propecia, will reduce the blood level of prostate-specific antigen (PSA). PSA is a serum marker that, when elevated, may be an indication of prostate cancer. Despite the fact that finasteride can alter PSA readings, do not be concerned that using it will compromise the accuracy of a PSA test. If you are taking finasteride, your doctor will make the necessary test adjustments.

Some additional information related to Proscar is equally reassuring. Millions of men have taken 5 milligrams of Proscar each day for ten years or more, and the drug has been generally well tolerated. In addition, finasteride hasn't displayed any negative drug interactions, which means it can be taken with other medication.

Risks for Women

Put simply, Propecia is not indicated for use in women. After conducting Phase III trials on the effects of finasteride on postmenopausal women, Merck concluded the drug was not effective in treating female androgenetic alopecia. Furthermore, when taken by pregnant women, finasteride can cause defects to the sexual organs of male fetuses. Pregnant women are further advised against handling pills that are broken or crushed, as there is a possibility that the drug can be absorbed through the skin and into the bloodstream.

Should a woman who is pregnant or trying to conceive have intercourse with a partner who is taking Propecia? Can the drug be transferred from the semen and absorbed through the vaginal wall? According to Merck, who conducted careful studies in this area, the amount of finasteride found in the average volume of ejaculate is so minute, there is no danger of transfer.

Dutasteride

As discussed earlier, there are two types of 5 α-reductase enzymes, Type I and Type II. Each converts testosterone into DHT, which causes hair loss. Finasteride blocks the formation of Type II DHT, while dutasteride blocks the formation of both types.

Developed by GlaxoSmithKline, dutasteride received FDA approval in 2002 for the treatment of benign prostatic hyperplasia (BPH) or enlarged prostate. Studies are in progress to see if, in fact, dutasteride's inhibition of both sources of DHT will result in either more hair growth or less hair loss than that seen with finasteride. So far, in preliminary studies, dutasteride has shown success in restoring hair to trial subjects. The details from these studies, including the range and severity of dutasteride's side effects, have yet to be published.

Dutasteride is not yet approved for the treatment of hair loss; however, physicians do have the option of prescribing it "off label" for treating male pattern baldness. This means that those who are willing to try this medication prior to FDA approval can do so by asking a physician for a prescription. Of course, this is done only with the understanding that it is being prescribed for nonapproved use. Before taking dutasteride, be sure to discuss the possible risks with your physician.

Antiandrogens

Antiandrogens are medications that block the function of male hormones. The antiandrogens spironolactone, flutamide, cyproterone acetate (not available in the United States), and gonadotrophin-releasing hormone analogues can effectively block increased levels of male hormones that cause hair loss in some women. Men who are experiencing androgenetic alopecia should never use these particular antiandrogens because of their side effects. In addition to significantly altering male hormone balance, these drugs also cause dimished sex drive and sexual function in men. Furthermore, androgenetic alopecia in men is not due to an *excess* of male hormones, but to the genetic predisposition of some follicles to normal levels of male hormones, which will cause their eventual loss. Women taking these medications may also experience side effects related to hormone level changes such as hot flashes, headaches, and vaginal dryness. Because of these side effects, the use of these medications is limited.

Ketoconazole is an antiandrogen that can be safely used by both men and women (those with excess male hormones). It is an antifungal antibiotic that is marketed in shampoo form to treat dandruff. Because it is applied to the scalp, ketoconazole is absorbed into the bloodstream in only minimal amounts, and, therefore, does not cause any untoward side effects. Nizoral brand shampoo containing a 1% solution of ketoconazole is available over-the-counter, while a 2% solution can be obtained by prescription. One study involving male subjects suggests that Nizoral 2% enlarges the hair shaft, and increases the percentage of hairs in the anagen growth phase. The effectiveness of this medication is similar to that received from 2% minoxidil. The study did not evaluate the impact on women's hair loss, but presumably, it would be effective only on females whose hair loss is due to excess male hormones, not androgenetic alopecia.

Women who exhibit signs of excess male hormones—excessive hair growth on the face or pubic area, infertility, and decreased or absent menstrual flow—should seek a medical evaluation in order to determine if an antiandrogen medication is appropriate. Laboratory tests can confirm the presence of elevated male hormones, and the appropriate medications can be prescribed. Ketoconazole appears to be a safe and easy-to-use treatment for hair loss, however the results obtained may be only modest at best.

Natural Treatments

The use of natural herbal remedies for the treatment of hair loss has become increasingly popular over the years. Claims of success have been made, but none of these treatments has had the benefit of undergoing a scientifically controlled study. Often these remedies are taken in conjunction with medications such as finasteride or minoxidil, making it difficult, if not impossible, to determine which part of the treatment may actually be beneficial. For your awareness, let's take a look at some of these natural treatments that are garnering attention.

Saw palmetto is sold as a natural remedy for prostate enlargement, and its benefits for this condition are supported by scientifically controlled studies. Because of its successful use for enlarged prostate, some have speculated that it may reduce DHT levels, much like finasteride. However, this has not been proven. In addition, there have been no studies showing saw palmetto's beneficial effects on hair growth, only anecdotal reports by individuals claiming success.

Other natural remedies that have been touted for their impact on hair loss include L-lysine, green tea, zinc, and grape seed extract. It has been established that a deficiency of L-lysine, an amino acid, will cause hair loss. Those who sell this product as a dietary supplement advertise this fact, hoping that it will cause consumers to infer that adding L-lysine to their diet will prevent or reverse hair loss. However, the only ones who would benefit from this treatment are those whose hair loss is specifically caused by an L-lysine deficiency, which is very rare.

Green tea, another so-called natural treatment for hair loss, contains *catechins*, a substance that has exhibited antiandrogenic properties. However, no studies have been done to examine the effectiveness of catechins in reversing hair loss. Studies have also indicated that high doses of zinc can inhibit the action of 5α-reductase, thus reducing levels of DHT. However, these studies were performed on laboratory animals, not human subjects. Grape seed extract contains an active ingredient that has been shown to prevent cellular damage, but offers little evidence that it can, in fact, grow hair.

Although these natural products may provide substances your body can utilize, or in some limited way, block the formation of DHT, their effectiveness in growing hair or preventing hair loss has never been proven in scientifically controlled studies. The choice to try these remedies is yours; however, don't be surprised if your expectations are not realized. If you do decide to try them, we strongly recommend discussing their use (or any other natural treatment) with your physician first.

CANDIDATES FOR PHARMACEUTICAL TREATMENTS

Nearly anyone with androgenetic alopecia who is bothered by hair loss can consider pharmaceutical options. Those in the early stages of hair loss are usually the best candidates. As explained earlier in this chapter, both minoxidil and finasteride work on the premise that some intermediate hairs can be influenced to regrow as terminal hairs. Those who have experienced the beginning stages of hair loss for a relatively short period of time are likely to have many intermediate hairs, which means they have a greater chance of finding these treatments effective.

Attitude is another important consideration in the decision to try pharmaceuticals. You must be both persistent and patient, willing to commit to using the products correctly for at least six months, and perhaps up to a year. No pharmaceutical hair-loss product can deliver instant results. The disappointment that some people experience when using these treatments is often due to their unrealistic expectations. For example, if a man with significant loss in the frontal and crown area (a Type IV or V pattern) starts the program expecting to maintain his current pattern, he is likely to be satisfied with the results. But if he begins to notice some new hair growth and then suddenly expects continued growth to transform him into someone with minimal loss (a Type II pattern), he'll be heading toward disappointment. Dissatisfied, he may decide to discontinue the treatment, which will cause him to start losing hair again.

Minoxidil and finasteride can stop hair loss in a significant number of men for a significant length of time. In some cases, they can even result in dense hair regrowth, but they cannot "cure" baldness. In addition, the ability to stop hair loss over the life of a person is unknown—the longest any study has examined success is five years. It is important to keep these limitations in mind.

Many men decide to try pharmaceutical options in addition to

If It Sounds Too Good To Be True . . .

"Finally, the cure is here! A revolutionary breakthrough product that is guaranteed to grow hair! No muss, no fuss, no adverse side effects. It's the answer to your prayers! Now anyone can reverse balding with 100% satisfaction!"

Of course, you've probably heard them all—the so-called "miracle" hair-growth products that are continually touted on television, in magazines, and on the Internet. Savvy marketers know just how to appeal to those who are experiencing hair loss and often desperate for that cure—that breakthrough cream or pill or special treatment that promises to reverse baldness and regrow lost hair.

Now hear this . . . no matter what you hear, no matter what a product promises, at this point in time, there is no "cure" for baldness. Other than minoxidil (the active ingredient in Rogaine), finasteride (found in the oral drug Propecia), dutasteride, and ketoconazole (found in Nizoral shampoo), no other drug or treatment has been scientifically proven to reverse, slow, or stop hair loss. And without legitimate, scientifically controlled studies, there is no way to verify a product's effectiveness.

In spite of this reality, so-called breakthrough products or treatments for "curing" hair loss continue to blaze their way into the marketplace, all claiming astonishing levels of success that are backed by "scientific research." But by investigating these too-good-to-be-true promises a little deeper, you'll discover that the products are not quite as "breakthrough" as the companies selling them would have you believe.

To begin with, many product studies claim dramatic positive results, but often fall into the category of "questionable" science. They were not conducted as controlled double-blind studies, and they were never published

surgery. This is a good idea and can be an effective way to handle your hair loss. The medication may help you keep the hair you have, while the surgery will add more hair to those areas in need. If you are undecided as to whether or not surgery is the right option for you, our recommendation is to start with the medication first, because the psychological value of having exhausted every avenue before undergoing surgery is enormous. Many of our patients have expressed feeling better about committing to surgery after they have tried a minoxidil product or Propecia. Futhermore, or peer-reviewed. In most cases, the company itself conducted the testing, which often involved only a single internal study.

Many products contain minoxidil, the active ingredient in Rogaine that has been legitimately tested and received FDA approval as an effective pharmaceutical for stimulating hair growth. However, in an effort to make their products seem unique, companies often add other ingredients to the minoxidil, which, they claim, makes their formulation "better." While these products may, in fact, show positive results, keep in mind that it is the minoxidil itself that is the cause. Considering these miracle solutions typically come with expensive price tags, remember that you are likely to do just as well with generic 2% minoxidil, which is less expensive and readily available.

Some companies actually mislead consumers by trying to hide the fact that minoxidil is the active ingredient in their product; it is listed on the label by its scientific name—2, 4-diamino-6-piperidino-pyrimidine-3-oxide. Even more disturbing, the companies boast that the ingredients in their formulas have been extensively tested with positive results. Of course, this statement is true, considering they are quoting the results of the minoxidil studies! And although they may claim the products have no known adverse side effects, the fine print warns to stop their use in the event of chest pain, accelerated heart beat, dizziness, swollen hands or feet, scalp redness or irritation, and unexplained weight gain—the same warning found on Rogaine and other minoxidil products.

So-called miracle hair-growth products will continue to flood the market as long as consumers maintain an "I'll-try-anything" mentality—companies rely on it. So *beware* of all the hype and misleading claims, and *be aware* of product reality. Think about it. If any of these incredible formulations really worked, why are there people out there who are still experiencing hair loss?

using the medication will give you more time to consider your hair loss, possibly allowing a fresh perspective. You may even decide to simply live with your hair loss.

Keep in mind that pharmaceuticals are specifically designed to combat androgenetic alopecia. They have not been proven effective in the treatment of other types of hair loss. (Although in rare cases, minoxidil may be used in the treatment of alopecia areata.) Anyone experiencing hair loss for any other reason should not use these products.

CONCLUSION

Pharmaceutical options are improving all the time. Perhaps one day soon, a new drug or therapy will be able to fully reverse the effects of male pattern baldness. But until that day, the existing proven medications can, in many cases, greatly reduce and/or delay hair loss, and may even regrow some hair. At the very least, they are an excellent means of giving you the time to think and calmly review other hair-replacement options. The importance of this cannot be overstated.

6

Surgical Options

"[We] should not expect something for nothing—
but we all do and call it Hope."

—EDGAR WATSON HOWE, COUNTRY TOWN SAYINGS

The surgical branch of hair replacement has grown significantly since the 1960s. The field has matured and transformed itself, and now offers some of the best options available for anyone who is interested in a permanent hair-loss solution.

After presenting some general guidelines that govern surgical hair rearrangement, this chapter takes a look at a variety of surgical options, including hair transplantation, alopecia reductions, and skin flap surgery. You will learn about each procedure, including its pros and cons. Following this important information, a section on what to expect throughout the surgical process—before, during, and after surgery—is presented. The chapter ends with an eye-opening discussion on bogus surgical procedures that you should be aware of and avoid.

THE LAW OF SUPPLY AND DEMAND

For the vast majority of patients—about 90 percent—surgical hair restoration involves a compromise. Of course, you could be one of the lucky few who is able to get exactly what you want, but it's not likely. So let's talk turkey about the unique nature of male pattern baldness, and the limitations of surgical hair rearrangement.

As you lose hair and the size of the bald area increases, the fringe area with hair decreases. In other words, as one area gets larger, the other shrinks. Because of this relationship, the law of supply and demand governs all hair-restoration surgery. Accordingly, a person can add only as much hair to the bald area (the demand) as can be provided by the fringe area (the supply). Any proposed plan for treatment that deviates from this fundamental principle is potentially damaging to your head. It can exhaust your donor supply before all of the bald areas are covered. You and your doctor must be extremely careful about how to use your precious donor hair.

A surgeon can use donor hair in two ways. He can either cut the hair-bearing skin from the fringe and literally move it, which is done during hair transplantation and when creating skin flaps; or he can stretch the hair-bearing skin so that it covers the bald area, which is what occurs during an alopecia reduction. Either way, only a finite amount of hair can be moved.

HAIR TRANSPLANTATION

The first hair transplant in the United States was performed in 1955 by Dr. Norman Orentreich in New York City. From that moment, the goal of surgical hair restoration has been the quest for achieving the greatest hair density while retaining complete undetectability and naturalness of appearance. Over the years, the technique of hair transplantation has been refined, and when done correctly, it is one of the best options for achieving naturalness, undetectability, and ease of styling and maintenance.

What Is a Hair Transplant?

Actually, there is no such thing as a hair transplant. What people commonly refer to as a hair transplant is actually a skin graft—a piece of skin that is taken from one part of the body and moved to another. During hair transplantation, that piece of skin just happens to contain hair follicles. It doesn't matter if the graft is the old "standard" 4-millimeter plug, a minigraft, a micrograft, or a follicular unit (all discussed later in this chapter)—all are considered skin grafts.

Regardless of a surgeon's preference in technique, all transplantation surgeries have certain common factors:

- They are "office procedures" that are performed in a doctor's office, not a hospital. They are also considered minor surgery—minor in comparison to "major" surgeries like heart transplants.

- Hair-bearing skin is cut from the back and/or sides of the fringe area of the head, known as the *donor area* or *donor site*. After this skin is removed, the surgeon will staple or sew the resulting wound shut.

- Grafts are cut from the large piece of hair-bearing skin, and then placed into small cuts or holes—called *recipient sites*—in the bald area. Hundreds, sometimes thousands of recipient sites will be made to accommodate the grafts. The grafts are gently grasped with surgical forceps (tweezers) or put into an automated inserter, and then placed into these sites. This is the method used for placing all types of grafts. In most cases, the bald area is located at the front and/or top of the head, but occasionally it is in the back or crown area—sometimes referred to as the *monk's spot.*

- The process of removing donor skin results in increased tension in the donor area and a progressively tighter scalp with each subsequent transplant procedure. Each time donor skin is harvested or removed, the density of the remaining hair in this area decreases. A tighter scalp and decreased hair density eventually conspire to end the surgeon's ability to safely remove any more donor skin. Nevertheless, even after repeated donor harvesting, the overall width or size of the fringe remains constant because of a phenomenon called *stretch-back,* which is explained later in the chapter.

Now that you are aware of hair-transplantation basics, it's time to discuss the various techniques.

Transplant Types

There are three basic types of grafting techniques used during hair transplantations. These include standard grafting, minigrafting/

micrografting, and follicular unit transplantation. Although standard grafting is rarely performed anymore, we discuss it here because it was the first type to be used.

Standard Grafting

When Dr. Orentreich discovered that "hair maintained the characteristics of the area from which it comes (the hair-bearing donor area), rather than to the area in which it is transplanted (the bald recipient area)," he coined this principle *donor dominance*. Based on this principle, he performed the first hair transplantation in 1955. During the procedure, he used what became known as a *standard grafting technique*. Standard grafts are round in shape, 4 millimeters in diameter (a little smaller than the size of a pencil eraser), and typically contain 16 to 20 hairs. Dr. Orentreich inserted the hair-bearing grafts into the bald area with a small punch, placing them about 1-graft size away from each other. This distance was to preserve the blood supply surrounding the newly placed grafts. In three subsequent sessions, which were spaced three to four months apart, he added more grafts in a "checkerboard" manner, as seen in Figure 6.1 below. Eventually, at the end of these sessions, the grafts touched or "kissed" each other, covering the bald area.

Dr. Orentreich's pioneering technique was truly a breakthrough in the field of hair restoration, but it wasn't without its drawbacks. Until the grafts had completely filled the bald area, their "plug-like" appearance was unsightly and easily detectable. Furthermore, because the grafts were large, the scarring they created was also more visible, rendering less than natural looking

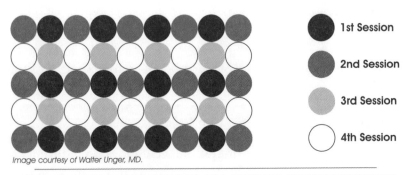

Image courtesy of Walter Unger, MD.

FIGURE 6.1. CHECKERBOARD PATTERN OF A STANDARD GRAFTING TECHNIQUE

results. Because of these drawbacks and the use of much-improved grafting methods, standard grafting is rarely used today.

Minigrafting / Micrografting

In 1981, Wayne Bradshaw, MD, a hair-restoration specialist from Perth, Australia, changed the traditional grafting process by using grafts that were much smaller than the standard type. His technique made transplanted hair less detectable than before, and is currently the most popular and frequently performed procedure in the world.

As indicated by its name, *mini/micrografting* is a technique that encompasses small grafts of different sizes—minigrafts and micrografts. A *minigraft* is usually square in shape, ranging in size from 1 to 2 millimeters, and containing 3 to 12 hairs. A *micrograft* is an even smaller graft that is 1 millimeter at best and usually contains no more than 2 hairs. While micrografts are critically important for the final result of a transplant to be natural in appearance, they may represent only a small percentage of the total number of grafts used in any single mini/micrograft session. *Slit-grafts* are a type of minigraft with 3 to 6 hairs, whose follicles are arranged in a line. Small slit-grafts contain 3 to 4 hairs; larger ones have 5 to 6.

All minigrafts and their recipient holes are "cut to size," which means the size of each graft matches the size of its recipient site. For any given amount of hair-bearing donor skin, any number of equal-sized minigrafts can be cut. Therefore, the larger the graft, the fewer that can be cut from the donor skin. But whatever the number is, the doctor will still be planting the same number of hairs into the same overall recipient area. However, the pattern or distribution of hair will change with the graft size. That is, the larger the graft, the fewer there will be to cover the given area. It also means that the distance from one graft to the next will be larger, as well. From a time- and cost-efficiency perspective, surgeons always want to cut and place as few grafts as possible. However, the larger the grafts and the farther apart they are placed, the greater the likelihood that they will be detectable and appear pluggy.

For each surgical session, the doctor will develop a plan to address the patient's needs. Based on this plan, which determines the type and number of grafts required, the appropriate amount of donor skin will be obtained. The surgeon will also determine the proper size of the recipient hole for each type of graft that is to be placed. He will then cut all of the recipient holes.

The number and types of grafts are then created from the donor skin with the aid of magnification and scalpel blades. Once created, the grafts are placed into the recipient sites. Typically, it takes three to five sessions to complete the transplantation process using mini/micrografts with anywhere from four to six months between sessions. Until the sessions are completed, there will be some degree of detectability.

The photographs in Figures 6.2 and 6.3 (below and on the facing page) are examples of hair transplants that were done using the mini/micrografting technique.

Follicular Unit Transplantation (FUT)

Considered by many as the "gold standard" of transplantation techniques, *follicular unit transplantation* (*FUT*) was pioneered in the early 1990s by Robert Limmer, MD, in San Antonio, Texas. In

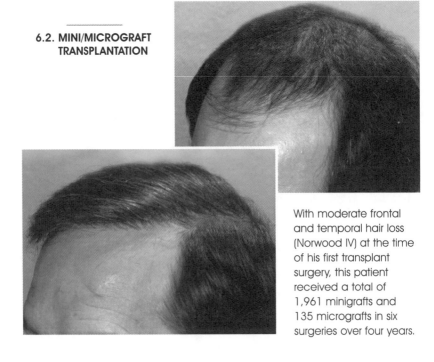

6.2. MINI/MICROGRAFT TRANSPLANTATION

With moderate frontal and temporal hair loss (Norwood IV) at the time of his first transplant surgery, this patient received a total of 1,961 minigrafts and 135 micrografts in six surgeries over four years.

1995, Robert Bernstein, MD, and William Rassman, MD, formalized the procedure when they published articles outlining the concepts, indications, and methodology of FUT. It is viewed as the best technique available for anyone desiring total undetectability, no matter how closely the hair is inspected.

Before describing this procedure, it's important to understand what a follicular unit is. For many years, most doctors believed that hairs grew individually and were spread out evenly over the entire head. But in 1984, J.T. Headington, MD, analyzed skin under a microscope and discovered that hair grew in discreet bundles or units, hence the term *follicular unit*. He observed that these units generally contain 1 to 4 hair follicles that are packed together and bound by collagen fibers. (See Figure 6.4 on page 98.)

Average Caucasian and Asian males have approximately 100 follicular units per square centimeter. Black men average 60 units. Hair density, however, does not solely depend on the number of units, but also on the number of hairs in each unit. To further explain, although Caucasian and Asian males each have about 100

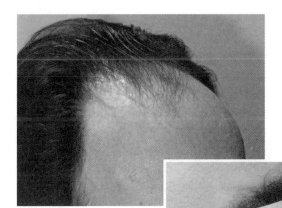

6.3. MINI/MICROGRAFT TRANSPLANTATION

At the time of his first surgery, this patient's hair loss extended beyond the midpoint of his scalp (Norwood IVa). Over a two-year period, he received 790 minigrafts and 575 micrografts in four surgeries.

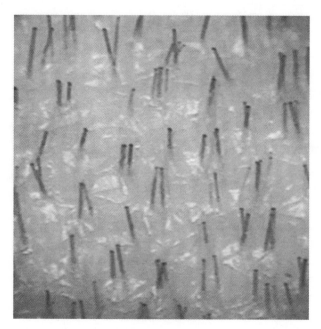

Follicular units on the surface of the scalp as seen through a microscope. Note the clustering of hair follicles into groups of 1, 2, 3, and 4 hairs. Also note the relatively large distance and the amount of "bald" skin between each unit.

Magnified view of individual follicular unit grafts that are ready for transplantation.

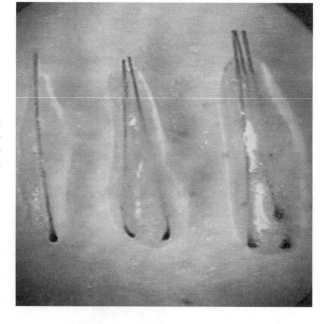

6.4. FOLLICULAR UNITS

follicular units per square centimeter, the number of hairs in each unit differs. For Caucasians, each unit contains approximately 2 hairs, which means 200 hairs per square centimeter. By contrast, the average Asian male, whose follicular units typically grow only 1 hair, have 100 hairs per square centimeter. Both men have the same number of follicular units, but because of the vast difference in the number of hairs, the density is not the same.

With the FUT technique, the surgeon or technician, with the aid of a microscope, makes the smallest grafts possible by separating the naturally occurring groupings of follicular units from the surrounding bald skin. Very small knife blades or hypodermic needles are used to create the recipient sites, which are much smaller than those made with the scalpels or punches used in minigrafting. By varying the angle and direction of the recipient site incisions, the doctor can control the growth pattern of the transplanted hair. It is the combination of the follicular units, the very small recipient sites, and the pattern of the grafts that allows FUT to mimic natural hair growth better than any other transplant technique. Complete undetectability, that is, hair that does not appear to be the result of a hair transplant, can be achieved.

Current advances in FUT include the isolation and extraction of a single follicular unit, which eliminates scars in the donor area and reduces healing time. Precise advantages and disadvantages of this new technique, however, have yet to be determined.

Follicular unit transplantation shares similar features with mini/micrografting. The process of obtaining the donor hair can be exactly the same, and the basic procedures are similar in that both require the creation and placement of the grafts. However, FUT is a longer procedure. Separating the follicular units, which is done with the aid of an operating microscope, is a timely process; also, the average number of grafts that are planted per session is higher. One minigraft, if separated into individual follicular units, can make anywhere from two to four grafts.

Using the microscope to create individual follicular units is what separates FUT from other hair-transplant procedures. This is important, as studies have shown that excessive damage occurs to follicles if a microscope is not used when preparing the grafts. An FUT surgeon and his or her staff typically implants anywhere from 800 to 3,000 grafts in a four- to eight-hour session.

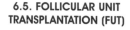

**6.5. FOLLICULAR UNIT
TRANSPLANTATION (FUT)**

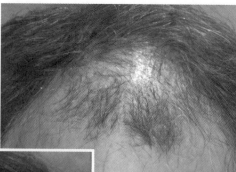

In a single session, this patient with significant hair loss (Norwood V), received 1,718 follicular unit grafts.

Even though very small incisions are made when creating recipient sites, there is still some trauma to the scalp. To limit this trauma and maintain adequate blood supply for growth, the grafts cannot be placed as close together as they were in the donor area. But this doesn't mean that FUT won't produce sufficient hair density. The human eye cannot tell the difference between the density of about 100 hairs per square centimeter and 200 hairs per square centimeter on the same man's head. In other words, by creating density that is 50 percent of the original, FUT can provide hair that visually matches normal hair density. However, it may take two or three sessions to achieve this.

Examples of hair transplants that were done using the FUT technique are displayed by the photographs in Figures 6.5 and 6.6 (above and on the facing page).

Hair Transplant Considerations

Hair-transplantation surgery has improved significantly since the

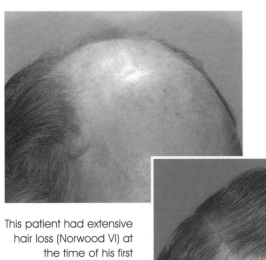

6.6. FOLLICULAR UNIT TRANSPLANTATION (FUT)

This patient had extensive hair loss (Norwood VI) at the time of his first transplant surgery. He received a total of 3,066 follicular unit grafts in two surgeries that were spaced nine months apart.

1990s. When done properly, the surgery can result in permanent natural-looking hair that is easy to style and maintain. Furthermore, with the advent of follicular unit transplantation, the surgical process can be completely undetectable from start to finish. Although mini/micrografting can be a great procedure, detectability is inevitable during the course of the treatments, and the final result will always be at least somewhat noticeable.

Transplants can be detectable for a wide range of reasons, including permanent skin color changes, scarring, and poor placement of the grafts. Most often, however, detectability refers to plugginess—grafts that are "pluggy" in appearance due to compression (discussed later in this chapter), or because they are simply too big, which is most common with standard grafting. Mini/ micrografting reduces these problems, and FUT eliminates them. Because FUT is undetectable from the very first surgical session, there is no pressure to have additional surgeries performed quickly to eliminate a pluggy or unnatural look. Younger men, whose final balding patterns cannot be determined, might choose to have one

FUT session, and then adopt a "wait and see" attitude for years, if necessary. They have time to evaluate their new hair and decide whether or not to add more. This is also a consideration for those individuals who cannot financially afford to complete the process quickly.

For most individuals, one of the biggest concerns about undergoing surgery is the healing time—how long the effects of the surgery will be noticeable. Follicular unit grafts take anywhere from four to nine days to appear totally normal—as if no surgery has taken place. Healing time after a minigraft or standard graft session is less predictable, usually taking anywhere from two to three weeks.

Of course, if done correctly, hair transplantation is permanent; your hair is your own and will remain so forever. You can comb it, style it, cut it—do anything you want to it—and it will remain. Maintenance and styling is easy. When making a decision on transplantation surgery, many men find this a highly motivating factor.

FUT, mini/micrografting, and even standard grafting can achieve excellent final density, but there are trade offs for each procedure. Standard grafting can produce high density in the recipient area, but the process is archaic, wasteful of donor hair, and detectable at all stages, often in the final result. Mini/micrografting can produce excellent final density, but the process itself is detectable. FUT produces a similar visual density as mini/micrografting, but does so with a much more efficient use of the donor supply, and it is never detectable. On average, both FUT and mini/micrografting require two or three sessions to produce good density. Some clinics can produce high-density FUT in a single session.

Dr. James Harris (coauthor of this book) has developed a variation of FUT for achieving hair density in a single session that would normally take two or three. The procedure is called *recombinant follicular unit transplantation*. This method involves the combination of follicular units (such as a 1-hair and a 3-hair unit), which are then *both* placed into a single recipient site. The size of the site is the same as it would be for a naturally occurring 4-hair unit. This "recombination" of follicular units allows each recipient site to have 3 or 4 hairs, unlike the standard FUT site, which has an average of 2 hairs. This procedure is intended for those over fifty years of age (the hair-loss pattern is usually better established) with limited hair loss and light or salt-and-pepper colored hair.

Proper Transplant Design

Proper aesthetic design and the location of grafts are the most important aspects of the transplantation process. Unfortunately, they are also the hardest to teach and learn.

The placement of the hairline is probably the single most important facet of proper hair-transplant design. If the hairline is improperly placed, the person receiving the transplant will simply not look right. The newly created hairline has to look "age appropriate." Generally speaking, the younger a man is, the lower and wider his hairline. Because of this, some people want their new hairline placed as low as possible with no recessions. Unfortunately, this doesn't work for most people, especially those who are older. With age, this type of hairline will do nothing more than make a person look "unusual."

Hairline placement is guided by the rule of thirds—the face can be divided into three similarly sized areas. The distance from the hairline to the eyebrow should measure the same distance as that from the eyebrow to the bottom of the nose, or from the bottom of the nose to the chin. Variations in facial structure also play a role in determining the placement and shape of the hairline. For example, a face that is triangular in shape tends to accentuate the forehead, while an elliptically shaped face is likely to minimize the same area. Hairline design should always compliment the person's face from both profile and frontal views.

In addition to the shape and location of the hairline, different "zones" are created by the way the different grafts are placed. A *density zone* on top of the head behind the frontal hairline will give the area a fuller, thicker appearance. Placing grafts with higher densities (3- and 4-hair units) in this area will create this zone. In the case of minigrafting, the larger grafts—those with more hair—are placed in this area to create the same effect.

The frontal hairline is not a "line" at all, but actually another zone. It is a *transition zone* that progresses from the bald forehead to the density zone immediately behind it. The transition zone is made of irregularly placed single-hair grafts in the first several rows, followed by 2-hair grafts in the area before the density zone begins. This grafting placement creates a soft, natural transition.

Another area that requires meticulous efforts in recreating a natural appearance is the crown, where a whorl or cowlick must be created. The progression of the cowlick in a spiral fashion with blending into the existing hair must have the proper graft direction and angle to appear normal. This area is very visible by someone standing behind or above the individual.

The recreation of these areas and zones requires attention to detail and skill. It is the natural appearance of these areas that will make the transplant undetectable to the casual observer.

Hair and Skin Characteristics

In addition to proper graft placement, other factors must be considered before transplantation, including the individual's hair and skin color combination, hair texture, and hair curl. Each of these factors will affect the outcome of surgery.

Nature has provided four natural camouflaging combinations of skin pigment and hair color that may render grafts less noticeable. These are red hair with a ruddy complexion; blond hair with fair skin; white, gray, or black-and-white (salt-and-pepper) hair with any skin color; and black hair with dark skin.

The most difficult hair-skin color combination for effective transplantation is a light skin tone with dark black or brown hair. The light skin acts as a background that actually highlights the space between grafts, making any plugginess more obvious. For those with this color combination, FUT may be the best option because it doesn't cause any plugginess. When mini/micrografting is used for those with this color combination, single hair grafts are usually placed in front of the larger grafts to help conceal the plugginess. People of Asian descent, whose skin is typically light and whose hair color is dark, often face this problem. Blacks, on the other hand, rarely have this color contrast problem, since their dark skin and hair often camouflage larger grafts very well.

In general, there are two dominant hair types—curly and coarse, and straight and finely textured. People with natural curl and coarse hair (large hair shafts) benefit from increased hair volume. Less hair is needed to cover larger areas of the bald scalp with no apparent decrease in density. For example, the average Black male has hair that is curly and coarse. When wearing his hair closely cropped, a great deal of scalp is exposed. But when his hair grows, it tends to look incredibly full. Each hair curls on itself, taking up more space and creating a convincing illusion of fullness. Individuals with straight, finely textured hair need more hairs per square centimeter to achieve similar volume.

The evaluation of the characteristics of hair color, curl, shaft thickness, and skin color should play an integral part during the consultation with a prospective surgeon. These factors will help guide the physician in projecting the potential surgical result and allow the patient to adjust his or her expectations accordingly.

Hair Transplant Risks

With rare exceptions, if a hair transplant doesn't work—the hair doesn't grow at all, it grows and then falls out, or it grows permanently in poorly selected places (such as a hairline that is placed too low)—it is due to the faulty technique of the surgeon. Unfortunately, many physicians entering this field believe that hair transplants are simple procedures. They don't understand the importance of proper aesthetics and the long-range planning that is required to achieve an undetectable, natural look for the rest of the person's life.

To further explain an error in long-range planning, take the example of transplanted hair that falls out after several years. This may happen if a surgeon incorrectly estimates future hair loss and takes grafts from an area that is too high in the fringe. Years later, if the patient has not stopped balding and the fringe has dropped below the line from where the grafts were taken, the grafts will lose hair as well. By not considering this potential future baldness, the doctor has erred in the long-range plans for his patient.

Regardless of the type of procedure, the surgical process of removing donor skin and cutting grafts will cause damage to a certain number of donor follicles. Potentially, standard and mini-grafting can damage about 20 percent of the follicles (some estimates are as high as 40 percent) if performed without microscopic dissection. FUT is least damaging, and when performed properly, can preserve over 95 percent of the donor follicles. The downside is that FUT is a very difficult, time-consuming, tedious technique, and many doctors simply do not perform it.

If you are interested in an FUT, be sure the surgeon is experienced and capable of performing this type of surgery. Putting your "head" in the hands of an inexperienced physician can put you at risk. Improperly done, this technique can result in problems with graft survival and the placement pattern. In other words, it is definitely better to have mini/micrografting performed by a skilled surgeon, than it is to have FUT done by an inexperienced surgeon who is struggling to learn the technique.

The Megasession

A *megasession* refers to a single surgery in which over 1,000 grafts are transplanted. The term typically refers to follicular unit transplantation, but it may also apply to a micrograft session that utilizes the same number of grafts. Some offices or clinics have the capability to transplant up to 3,000 grafts in one session. Megasessions do have their advantages. Specifically, they cover larger areas than smaller sessions do. This means fewer surgeries are required. When fewer grafts are used, more sessions are necessary to achieve the same density and coverage that can be achieved in a megasession. Fewer sessions mean less overall "down time" recovering from the procedures.

If the initial surgery involved a sufficient number of grafts and was performed properly, the person can decide to stop at any time with a look that is natural and undetectable. Subsequent sessions can be planned to increase the density in an area that has been previously transplanted, or to focus on another balding area. We always recommend that you give yourself more options and flexibility when possible, which means waiting the appropriate amount of time between procedures.

Hair Transplantation for Women

The treatment of women's hair loss requires its own approach. Unlike men, women rarely lose all of the hair in an affected area. Often, much of the hair remains, but the shafts become thinner, resulting in areas of meager volume. Transplantation involves placing hair into a part of the scalp that is thinly covered, but not completely bald. The existing hair in this area is at risk, as it may be damaged or lost because of the transplantation. In addition, if the donor area continues to thin, the transplanted hair will also thin over time, since it came from the same area. Because a relatively large area can be subject to thinning, it is not possible to transplant the entire scalp; there is not enough donor area to meet the demand. It is important that hair is transplanted in the most appropriate spots—either where it is cosmetically most significant, or where it can enhance a specifically defined styling plan. For example, in some cases, the grafts may be confined to a localized area of the scalp, such as behind the frontal hairline or "along the part." And if a woman has a dense donor area that does not appear to be subject to thinning or loss, it may be possible to provide more coverage over the top of her scalp.

To successfully perform hair transplantation in women, the surgeon must understand the subtle, but important, aesthetic differences between the sexes. A normal female hairline is much different from a male's, often characterized by abrupt directional hair changes, which give the frontal edge its character. These whorls or cowlicks can be recreated, but require great attention to the depth, angle, and spacing of the recipient sites.

Some female hairlines have another interesting characteristic known as a *widow's peak*—a V-shaped point that is formed by the hair in the middle of the forehead. The widow's peak is not simply a triangular dip at the midline, but a series of variations in the hairline that can be both dramatic and elegant. The peak is often bounded on at least one side by a concave rather than a convex hairline. It is often slightly off center and asymmetrical. Also, the hair of the peak often points to the side.

Because the female hairline is characteristically irregular and often asymmetric, a good surgeon must fight his instincts to be orderly when determining the placement of the grafts. If the grafts are too organized, they won't look natural. The surgeon must, therefore, possess the knowledge, experience, and foresight to strike just the right blend of asymmetry and irregularity with balance and precision.

Any female who is considering transplantation should feel comfortable with her choice of surgeon. This doctor should be experienced in performing successful hair transplants on women.

Hair Transplant Candidates

About 99 percent of all balding and bald men, regardless of their degree of hair loss, are perfectly acceptable candidates for hair transplantation. There are, however, a few prerequisites that should be met to help ensure success.

First, anyone considering hair transplantation must understand the supply-and-demand limitations imposed by their own balding patterns. The most important quality that a prospective candidate can possess is a realistic expectation. This outweighs all other factors. Those who desire complete elimination of every centimeter of baldness with high uniform density in all transplanted areas are unrealistic; they're not likely to be happy with transplantation. Long-time hair addition wearers in particular have difficulty accepting and adjusting to the look and feel of transplanted coverage, because it is simply not as thick as a hair addition.

Good general health is another surgical prerequisite. Although hair transplantation is considered minor surgery, it is still invasive and, therefore, carries potential risks. When filled out completely and honestly, a medical history form will alert the doctor to allergies, prior surgeries, emotional problems, medical conditions, and the pertinent family history of prospective patients. If you are currently under a doctor's care for any illness, the transplant surgeon should contact your doctor and discuss the procedure in relation to your particular condition. There are very few medical conditions that prevent hair-rearrangement surgery. Nevertheless, honesty on the patient's part and thoroughness on the part of the doctor is always the wisest policy.

As for age, there is no ideal or correct time in one's life for hair transplantation. While there are no hard and fast rules, and every case should be evaluated individually, men who are under age twenty-five are generally not good candidates. They are just beginning to lose their hair and starting to develop a mature male hairline. It is not uncommon for a twenty-five-year old to see the maturation of his hairline and desire that it be "corrected" to look like it did at age eighteen. However, this correction would not be appropriate because the resulting hairline will be too low or wide when the man is in his forties or fifties. Another reason it isn't advisable to perform transplantation on a man of this age is because the future extent of his hair loss is unknown, making it difficult, if not impossible, to manage the supply of his hair to the eventual demand.

In general, the older one is, the more accurately a surgeon can estimate the extent of hair loss and formulate a long-term plan for use of the available donor hair. This maximizes the chances of achieving a natural-looking result that will last for the rest of the person's life.

There is also no amount of male pattern hair loss that precludes surgery, provided the patient is aware of the law of supply and demand. In other words, he can get only as much coverage as the donor supply allows.

Patient expectations also play a role in determining a good candidate for surgical hair restoration of any type. For example, a patient must be aware that transplanting standard grafts and minigrafts requires a long-term commitment to treatment that includes an average of three to five surgeries. During that period, detectability is always a concern and the transplant candidate has to be emotionally prepared for it. Minigrafting requires a minimum of three sessions to achieve a satisfactory level of undetectability and natural appearance if the person is starting with a totally bald area. FUT, however, eliminates this concern because it results in a natural look after only one session. Even with FUT, the expectations must be realistic as a "natural" appearance is different from a "dense" appearance. Of course, if a patient desires greater density and/or more coverage, additional sessions will be necessary for either procedure. The point here is that the patient should have a reasonable idea of what to expect from any procedure.

One final and very important factor that must be considered as a prerequisite to hair transplantation is the *cause* of one's baldness. The vast majority of men who have male pattern baldness, which is also the most common type, can enjoy success with transplantation surgery. People whose hair loss is caused by scars from an accident or trauma are also excellent candidates. The follicular units can be placed into the scar tissue, resulting in good coverage of the area. Often, this not only provides cosmetic benefits, but may also ease some of the emotional stress caused by the scarring. Other causes of hair loss, such as the scarring alopecias, may not be amenable to transplantation. As discussed in Chapter 3, women must be evaluated for causes of hair loss before any surgical treatment is considered. If a medical reason is found, the treatment must be directed at the cause.

Transplant Cost

The cost of a hair transplant procedure can depend on many factors. The most basic is the price that a physician will charge per graft, whether it's a follicular unit, minigraft, or standard graft. Other factors include the area of bald scalp to be covered (more area means more grafts) and the patient's desire for density (greater density means more grafts). The variability between costs from office to office is usually due to regional differences in overhead expenses and competition.

Follicular unit transplantation ranges from $3.00 to $12.00 per graft while mini/micrografts and standard grafts range from $3.00 to $15.00 per graft. Keep in mind that although the price may be similar between follicular unit grafts and minigrafts, the number of grafts placed in a FUT session, will, on average, be higher. Some doctors will charge a flat fee for a session of mini/micrografts, which can range from $3,000 to $10,000. The most effective way to compare costs is by speaking to the surgeon and obtaining an estimate of the total number of hairs that are to be transplanted, and then calculating the cost per hair. This may be the only way to compare costs between the different surgical techniques, but just keep in mind that it is a highly subjective method and prone to inaccuracies.

ALOPECIA REDUCTIONS

Although hair-rearrangement techniques have certainly improved over the years, all transplants are governed by—and limited by—the law of supply and demand. A person can add only as much hair to the bald area as can be provided by the donor area. Often, hair grafts are limited to the front half of the bald scalp, because there simply may not be enough donor hair to cover other areas as well. Understandably, patients constantly ask, "Can't I have some more hair? Can't we go further back?"

During the mid-1970s, when standard grafts were being used, several doctors theorized that with less bald area, the same number of grafts could provide greater coverage. Their idea was to remove some of the bald area so that fewer grafts from the precious, irreplaceable donor supply would be needed to cover the hairless area. Brilliant, right? Well, not exactly.

What Is an Alopecia Reduction?

Alopecia reductions (AR), commonly referred to as *scalp reductions*, are procedures that reduce the area of bald skin. For a number of reasons, they are not performed as frequently as they were in the past.

Considered minor surgery, alopecia reductions are performed in the doctor's office, although they are more involved than most hair transplants. During this procedure, an area of bald scalp is cut and removed. The pattern in which the scalp is cut is commonly in the shape of an inverted "Y" (like the Mercedes Benz logo) or an "S." The pattern is chosen to minimize detectability of the scar or to best suit the surgeon's plan for subsequent surgery. The remaining skin on both sides of the exposed wound is then stretched over the area and sutured or stapled together. This stretching results in an overall increase in scalp tension. Because the fringe or donor area is also stretched, the hair density in this area is decreased. The scar from this procedure is located either in the middle of the bald area or at the top edge of the fringe, but it is never totally hidden. After an alopecia reduction, the bald area will be smaller in size. It will also have visible scars, which, in most cases, are camouflaged with grafts.

A number of devices and procedures have been developed to augment alopecia reductions by stretching the hair-bearing skin. The theory is that if you can "create" more hairy skin, then theoretically, you can remove more bald scalp. Scalp expanders, scalp extenders, and extensive scalp lifting are all intended to increase the amount of "hairy" skin to further cover the bald area. Of course these techniques only stretch the hair-bearing skin; the total amount of potential donor hair remains the same.

A *scalp expander* is a silicone balloon that is placed under the hair-bearing scalp. It is slowly filled with sterile water over a period of six to ten weeks for the purpose of stretching the skin. This area, which is covered with hair, will replace the bald area that has been removed during the alopecia reduction. Using the scalp expander actually involves two surgeries. During the first surgery, the balloon device is placed under the skin. After the skin has been expanded and stretched, a second surgery is required to remove the device. During this second surgery, the alopecia reduction will also be performed.

As the balloon enlarges during the scalp expansion process, an obvious cosmetic deformity occurs. Because of this and because the surgical alternatives for hair replacement have evolved to the point where there is little or no detectability, most men are not interested in this option. It is reserved for the reconstruction of victims with extensive scarring from traumatic injuries or burns.

Various types of *scalp extenders*, which are placed under the bald skin but whose ends are "hooked" to the hairy fringe, apply slow, constant tension to stretch the fringe. Once the area is stretched, which may take thirty to forty days, it is used to cover the portion of bald skin that has been removed during the alopecia reduction. This is a two-step procedure. The first step involves inserting the extender; the second step, which is performed during the alopecia reduction, involves removing the extender, and then replacing part of the bald area with the stretched skin. The stretched portion is always adjacent to the bald area that's being cut away. When the extender is removed, the skin is bunched up like the wrinkled skin of a Sharpei dog. It is then flattened and used to cover the area. This method can be quite painful because the scalp is under a great deal of tension.

The procedure called *extensive scalp lifting* uses *undermining*—a process that separates the hair-bearing skin from the deeper layers of tissue. This creates an entire fringe area of skin with hair that is separated from the skull and upper neck. As the bald skin is removed from the top of the head during the reduction, the loose skin is then pulled towards the top of the scalp, redraped, and sewn into place. The undermining begins at an incision that is made just above the fringe, and then extends under the entire fringe from ear to ear, down the back of the head and into the neck area, sometimes to the collar bone. Once the skin is separated from the deeper tissues, it is redraped as just described. The purpose of this procedure is to reduce the bald area without stretching the fringe area.

Because the popularity of alopecia reductions has declined, the use of these adjunctive techniques has declined as well. Under certain circumstances, these procedures can play a helpful role in hair-rearrangement surgery, but not for the average person with androgenetic alopecia.

Considerations of Alopecia Reductions

Alopecia reductions can dramatically aid in the repair and reconstruction of areas of scarring that have resulted from disease (skin tumors), accidents (lacerations, burns, etc.), or poor cosmetic surgery. Large scarred areas can be removed in this relatively minor procedure. As a matter of fact, these conditions are the only indications for alopecia reduction in women. Its use for reducing baldness is its least important objective; however, from a very limited perspective, the cosmetic improvement attained with alopecia reduction surgery is dramatic and instantaneous. But at what price? Read on.

Problems with Alopecia Reductions

Fewer alopecia reductions are performed today than ever before. The general consensus among surgeons is that they are simply not the fix-all procedures they were once believed to be. We agree, firmly believing that alopecia reductions should be used only for reconstructive surgery, not for cosmetic enhancement.

Although the major goal of an alopecia reduction—reducing the size of the bald area—may appear to be a positive step for those interested in hair transplantation, the procedure has inherent risks and pitfalls. The most apparent problems include the following:

- **Reduced Density and Scalp Laxity**
By stretching the hair-bearing scalp to cover the area where bald skin has been removed, alopecia reductions decrease hair density

in the fringe. Plus, they stretch the fringe, creating a tighter scalp. These two factors significantly diminish the ability of the fringe to act as the donor supply. Even though the same amount of donor hair still exists, the tighter scalp prevents its removal. Why? When a strip of hair-bearing hair is removed from the fringe, the surrounding skin must have enough elasticity and "looseness" so the resulting wound can be sewn closed.

• Inadequate Coverage
Alopecia reductions do little to increase hair where it's cosmetically most important—on the front portion of the scalp. As this procedure reduces bald areas by lifting the fringe area higher, it is the back and side portions of the head that gain the most hair.

• Stretch-Back
Skin contains collagen and elastin fibers that react to the reduction by stretching and extending. As the skin stretches, the scar and bald area get larger than they were just after the surgery. If you hike up the fringe, it stretches back. Hike it up some more, it stretches back again, until finally, the scalp is totally "stretched out."

• Slot Deformation and White Sidewalls
In an attempt to decrease the problem of stretch-back, some surgeons recommend undermining (discussed on page 112), which enables a surgeon to move the hair-bearing fringe to the top of the head. Although this can be effective in combating stretch-back, it gives rise to two new problems. First, the hair that is now on the top of the head is misdirected. Instead of pointing forward on the top of the head, it points towards the ears. A second resulting problem is *slot deformation*—a scar that runs down the center of the head, caused by the joining of the two fringes. Some people are able to comb the hair over the slot deformation, but for many, the hair flops back to its original position, exposing the scar.

Another major problem with undermining is that it raises the hairline at the bottom of the fringe abnormally high, causing *white sidewalls*—exposed skin (sometimes several inches) above the ear. The only solution, besides growing the hair long, is transplanting hair in the area to lower the hairline. This, however, wastes grafts that could be used in the front of the head.

• **Scarring**

Alopecia reductions leave scars *100 percent* of the time. The scars will vary in size and shape depending on how that particular person heals—and people do heal differently. If you took 100 men and made an incision down the middle of their bald heads (even if you didn't remove any skin), the resulting scars would vary in shape and dimension. Scars heal with the aid of collagen fibers, which contract over time. The slightest contraction on a bald scalp will cause a reflection of light that is different from the surrounding skin. Even if the scar is as thin as a pencil tip, it will be noticeable.

• **Halo Formation**

Although covering a scar with transplanted hair is an option, it does have its downside. First, it uses up precious grafts. Second, for the person with a moderate degree of baldness, a *halo formation* is likely to occur around the grafted area. As the individual continues to lose hair, which statistically he will, the fringe will begin to separate from the hair-covered scar, surrounding it with a halo of bare skin. It will look like a spreading sea of baldness encircling an island of hair.

The doctor will be committed to filling in the halo area for as long as the patient continues to bald—a process known as *chasing the fringe*. Most distressing is that the doctor will be using grafts that could be better used elsewhere on the person's head. Instead of transplanting hair into the halo of baldness, the surgeon *could* suggest another reduction to remove this bald area, but that would only result in more scars. Furthermore, additional transplants will be needed to cover the new scars.

Considering the effective results that can be obtained with the current hair-transplant options and the wide range of problems that can result from an alopecia reduction, it is apparent that a reduction is not the optimal choice. Before deciding on this type of procedure, be sure you are aware of all of its possible downsides, and be certain your physician can correct any resulting problems.

Cost

Fees for an alopecia reduction range from $3,000 to $9,000. The more complicated procedures involving the use of expanders and extenders are more expensive because they require greater technical skills, the devices themselves, and multiple office visits.

SKIN FLAPS

Skin flaps were developed in 1969 by Dr. Jose Juri in direct response to standard grafting, which often had poor results. The procedure involves moving a relatively large piece of hair-bearing skin to a bald area, while one side of this skin remains attached to the original blood supply.

There are several types of flaps that differ according to their length and the location from where they are obtained. Basically, skin flap surgery is a four-step procedure that is performed over the course of three to four weeks. The hair-bearing skin on the side of the head is transferred to the frontal area or mid-scalp region where a similarly sized piece of bald skin is removed to make room for the flap. The area in the hair-bearing fringe that is left open by the removal of the flap is stretched and sewn together. The existing hair completely hides the scar.

Considerations of Skin Flaps

Skin flaps have several positive aspects. They address the problem of plugginess, since no individual grafts are moved and planted. When the flaps are moved, they do not cause shock loss (discussed in Chapter 3) that may be caused by grafting. Flaps also provide instant gratification. Instead of multiple surgeries and months of waiting for hair to grow, a single flap surgery can provide thick normal hair in the bald area in one day. Once healing is complete, in one to two weeks, the hair should continue to grow as it did in its original location.

Problems with Skin Flaps

There are several significant problems with most skin flaps. To begin with, there is the abruptness of the hairline. Unless the surgeon plants follicular unit grafts in the area in front of the flap to ensure a natural transition, flap hairlines are always detectable.

Another possible problem is *tip death,* in which the tip or end of the flap dies due to insufficient blood. Proper technique plays a crucial role in preventing this, but it can happen with even the best surgeons. When tip death occurs, the dead area must be replaced with a patch of the surrounding hair-bearing skin. Sometimes, an entire flap dies, although this is extremely rare.

And then there's the problem with the flap's hair direction, which literally points 180 degrees in the wrong direction. Normally, hair on the front of the head grows from the scalp at a slight forward angle. Flap hair, because of its source in the fringe near the ears, grows in a direction towards the crown and back of the head. Men who wear their hair combed straight back will have no problem with flaps. But those who want their hair to fall forward onto the forehead will be seriously frustrated.

Exposed scars along the front edge of the flap are hard to camouflage—often because they are a different color, usually lighter, than the forehead skin. Fortunately, follicular units transplants can help make a great difference, but they can't guarantee complete scar undetectability.

Also, flaps are restricted in the type of hairline they can create. The shape tends to reflect one of pre-adolescence, not one of a fifty-year-old male. With flaps, it is difficult to create the temporal recessions that reflect the normal aging and thinning process that most men experience. Secondary surgeries may be required to adjust the shape of the hairline and to add recessions. Unfortunately, even after additional surgery, flap hairlines still look unnatural to some degree.

The hair created by many flaps is too thick to appear normal over the patient's lifetime. As a man continues to bald, the unnatural density of the flap hair will contrast with the lesser density of hair in the mid-scalp region, highlighting the fact that he has had surgery.

Who Should Consider Flaps?

People who have naturally rounded hairlines and people with very curly hair are good candidates for flap surgery. Blacks tend to have both of these characteristics, and, therefore, can find natural results using flaps. The other type of individual who may benefit from flaps would be a Caucasian or Asian male with a stable balding pattern of Norwood Type IV (moderate thinning of the frontal scalp area, as seen in the chart on page 51), is over the age of forty-five, and is very concerned about density. Naturally curly hair will further serve to camouflage the problems with hair direction and abrupt hairlines.

Cost

Skin flap procedures usually cost somewhere in the range of $4,000 to $10,000. The fee typically depends on the size and number of flaps, as well as the surgeon's skill and experience.

Although skin flaps can result in areas of high hair density, as you have seen, their problems are numerous. They are not indicated for the average person.

THE SURGICAL PROCESS

Although it is not complicated, the surgical process involved with hair rearrangement involves much more than simply showing up on the day of surgery. By following some simple guidelines before, during, and after surgery, you will find that you can do much to minimize stress, maximize comfort, and avoid complications that can compromise success.

Before Surgery

To help ensure that the day of your surgery runs smoothly, your surgeon will give you some presurgical instructions to follow. Typically, these preparations will begin a few weeks prior to the procedure.

If the doctor plans on obtaining any lab work, including tests for bleeding and clotting disorders, hepatitis, and HIV, this should be completed about two to three weeks before surgery. Your doctor will also provide you with a list of drugs, herbal treatments, and vitamins that should be avoided because they can disrupt the body's blood-clotting mechanism. For instance, vitamin E should be avoided for two weeks prior to the procedure, while aspirin and aspirin-containing products should not be used during the week before. And if you use Rogaine or other minoxidil product, stop using it for the entire week before surgery. Don't use alcohol, unapproved drugs, or marijuana for forty-eight hours prior to the transplantation. These substances can interfere with the body's blood-clotting process and increase the amount of bleeding during the surgery.

On the other hand, some studies indicate that vitamin C may speed the healing process, so your doctor may advise you to begin taking 2,000 milligrams per day, starting one week prior to the procedure. Your surgeon will review any medications you are taking and advise you on whether or not they should be discontinued. Most doctors will prescribe antibiotics to begin taking the day before surgery to help prevent post-operative infection.

For maximum coverage in the donor area, we encourage you to let your existing hair grow to at least one inch in length. Wash your hair well either the night before or on the morning of the procedure. Do not use hair conditioners, which contain oil or wax that attracts dirt. Finally, try to get at least eight hours of sleep the night before the procedure.

It is not unusual to experience presurgical anxiety in varying degrees. For the majority of people, the antidote to anxiety before surgery is information. A quick call to the office to review information, ask a question, or address a concern can often quell those jitters. Some individuals need to meet with patients who have just had the surgery and are returning to the office for a post-op cleanup. If you are feeling anxious and none of these efforts has helped to put you at ease, don't hesitate to ask your doctor for a mild sedative or sleeping pill to take the night before the procedure. A sleepless night will only make you more anxious.

The Day of Surgery

The day of surgery should be a calm one. Most people find that an understanding of what is likely to occur on this day—before, during, and after the procedure—helps insure peace of mind.

Before Arriving at the Office

Before having most types of surgery involving grafting techniques, be sure to have a light breakfast or lunch. This will help keep your blood sugar level from dropping too low during the procedure, which can cause fainting. Acceptable foods include dry toast, soft-boiled eggs, juice, clear broth, skim milk, and decaffeinated coffee or tea. Forego anything that is fried or covered in butter, cheese, or cream. If you are having an alopecia reduction or a flap procedure, the doctor may recommend that you avoid eating anything after midnight the night before the surgery. Eating may increase the chances of nausea and vomiting, which can increase the risk of complications.

Once at the office, you will have to remove your shirt and shoes, and put on a patient gown. For this reason, be sure to wear clothes that are easy to remove and put back on. Button type shirts and shoes like loafers or sneakers are recommended. Putting on a pullover shirt after surgery can dislodge grafts, and straining to take off or put on boots can elevate blood pressure, which may cause bleeding.

Pre-Operative Sedation

To help ensure a positive surgical experience, we recommend pre-operative sedation to help you relax before the local anesthetic is administered. Not all surgeons, however, give sedation as a standard practice.

There are three main forms of pre-operative sedatives—nitrous oxide (gas), oral medication (pills), and intravenous (IV) medications. Breathing nitrous oxide, which you may have had at the dentist's office, brings about a sense of relaxation and calm. Pills fall into two categories—anti-anxiety and analgesics. The most commonly used oral medications for anti-anxiety include Valium, Xanax, Halcion, and Dalmane. Versed and Valium are the anti-anxiety medications that are typically given intravenously. Analgesics for pain relief include drugs like Tylenol with codeine, Percocet, and Darvocet. The medications just mentioned are sometimes used in combination to achieve specific pain relief and anti-anxiety effects.

If you don't like the idea of intravenous medication and prefer pills, that's fine. Just be sure to arrive early enough to allow the medication the time it needs to take effect. Valium and Percocet tablets, for instance, take about forty-five minutes to "kick in." If you swallow them as you're walking down the hall to the operating room, it will be totally ineffective during the surgery. Over the years, we have had patients who were intensely interested in every aspect of the surgery and wanted to be as wide-awake as possible during the procedure. They didn't want any pre-operative sedation, opting instead to endure the occasional twinge for the few minutes that it took to numb the donor and recipient areas. If you are one of these patients, go for it. The key to a pleasant experience, tailored precisely to your needs, is honest and open communication with your doctor and his or her staff.

The number-one side effect of pre-operative medications is drowsiness, which occurs in differing degrees among individuals, and is impossible to determine in advance. Some patients even complain of feeling very drowsy the morning following the surgery. For them, adjustments in the medication can be made prior to subsequent surgeries.

Finally, if you are going to receive a sedative before your procedure, arrange to have a friend or family member take you home. If this isn't possible, be sure to make plans for car service.

The Photographs

At some point prior to surgery, you will be photographed from several different angles to document the degree of your hair loss. Photos should be taken before each and every procedure.

The Procedure

Just before beginning the actual procedure, the surgeon will draw guidelines on your head with a special marker. For reductions and flaps, an incision pattern will be drawn. For transplants, a hairline and/or the areas that are to be filled with grafts will be marked. As this is being done, the surgeon should once again review the plan for the procedure with you. The hair on the donor area of the scalp will then be clipped.

Once in the operating room, you will be placed on a surgical table or seated in a surgical chair, depending on the type of procedure and the preference of the surgeon. At this point, the doctor may administer a sedative intravenously to achieve a "twilight sleep"—that hazy stage between full awareness and deep sleep. Once you are properly sedated, the surgeon will numb the main nerve centers of the scalp, using an anesthetic that is similar to the one you receive for dental surgery. For most patients, this is the most dreaded part of the procedure because the anesthesia is injected directly into the skin. What's most important is getting the area numb with minimal pain and discomfort. Fortunately, this is both possible and quite simple.

You, and *only* you, should control the "numbing" phase of the surgery. We cannot overstate this point. Because the injections should be nearly painless, they are given as slowly or as quickly as you want. Only *you* know if something hurts; therefore, only you can tell the surgeon to slow down. The right amount of time to accomplish this phase of the procedure is however long it takes to numb your head painlessly. It takes less than five minutes to numb some patients and more than twenty-five to anesthetize others. Remember, the doctor who cares about your comfort level will also care about your final appearance.

During the surgery, if you begin to feel the numbness wearing off, tell someone immediately. A small percentage of people are "rapid metabolizers"; their anesthesia wears off faster than it does for the average person. It is your right to be completely numb throughout the entire procedure, but it is also your responsibility to speak up. After all, the surgeon has no way of knowing what you're feeling.

After Surgery

After the procedure, your most immediate concern will probably be dealing with any pain you may feel as the anesthesia wears off. Fortunately, there is much you can do to relieve postsurgical pain and avoid postsurgical complications.

Pain Control

After surgery, you will be given written instructions for the following week. Your doctor may give you two or three sleeping pills to help you rest comfortably during the first few nights after surgery. Transplant patients rarely, if ever, feel pain in the recipient area where the grafts have been placed. They do, however, complain of discomfort in the donor area, especially since their heads rest on the suture line during sleep. The pain in this area, which usually doesn't last longer than forty-eight hours, may require a mild narcotic.

The first option for controlling this type of pain is Marcaine, a local anesthetic that can be injected into the donor area just before leaving the office. It will keep the incision site pain free for five to six hours. Your doctor may also give you a packet of pain pills, ranging from basic Tylenol to more serious painkillers such as Darvocet, Vicodin, or Percocet. There is no reason to endure pain. Take a pill even if you only imagine that you might be experiencing pain. You're only going to need painkillers for one or two nights at most. *Do not take any pain medications containing aspirin, as this can interfere with blood clotting.*

It is in your best interest to discuss pain relief with your doctor prior to the day of surgery, and to be sure that you are in agreement with the plan. Remember, you have an absolute right to expect and receive the best medication that can be provided for the control of pain and discomfort.

The Post-Operative Checkup

The post-operative checkup is usually scheduled the morning after surgery. Implanted grafts must be checked to make sure that they haven't dislodged. Any suture lines from an alopecia reduction, a skin flap, or from hair removal in the donor area, must be inspected for oozing, unusual swelling, and discoloration. After this examination, any area of your head that was directly affected by the surgery will be washed, and if your hair is long enough, it will be styled to cover any noticeable surgical wounds.

The most frequently asked question regarding the surgery is, "How will I look to others?" The answer depends upon your degree of hair loss, as well as how important you feel it is to conceal your surgery. The simplest way to cover transplanted sites is by wearing a loose-fitting ventilated cap, such as a baseball or golf cap. If you'd rather not wear one, combing your existing hair (provided it's long enough) over the graft sites is an option. Do not wear a hair addition for at least the first thirty-six hours after surgery. After that, a hair addition should not be worn longer than two to three hours at a time. It is also best if the hair addition has a mesh base that allows for ventilation. The surgical wounds should be kept dry, except during the usual bathing. As for the donor site, the surrounding hair will keep any incisions easily concealed.

Other Postsurgical Expections

If you have had minigrafts, micrografts, or a follicular unit trans-plant, expect the grafts to form crusts or scabs within the first three days. Varying in thickness from 1 to 3 millimeters, these crusts may cause the minigrafts to appear elevated from the surrounding skin, but when they drop off two to three weeks later, properly trans-planted minigrafts will be smooth and flush to the scalp. All of the crusts on micrografts or follicular unit grafts typically fall off in four to nine days. Regular washing and shampooing, plus the use of an antibacterial ointment, can help them come off sooner. Scab-bing along suture lines in the donor area or on scalp incisions from alopecia reductions or flaps should be gone within three weeks. Never pick at an incision; allow the crusts to fall off naturally.

Approximately one week after surgery, any nondissolvable sutures, including stainless steel surgical staples, can be removed. If you have traveled a long distance for the surgery, you might choose to have a local doctor remove the sutures. Some surgeons use dissolvable sutures that fall off by themselves, eliminating the need to return to the office.

Caring for Grafts and Incisions

After a hair-transplantation session, bandages are simply not nec-essary. However, after an alopecia reduction or flap surgery, the incisions will be bandaged. During the post-operative checkup, the bandages will be removed. Do not take them off yourself for any reason.

After undergoing any hair-rearrangement procedure, try to keep your head exposed to the air for the first seven to ten days to aid healing. Avoid wearing a hat or hairpiece whenever possi-ble. Although you can expose your head to the sun, be careful to avoid sunburn. You may also experience some dandruff-like scal-ing, redness, or itching during the first month after the procedure. Apply hydrocortisone cream or lotion to the affected area two to four times daily until the itching is gone.

Do not massage or manipulate the scalp for any reason! You can rupture the healing skin and prolong the healing process. This can also cause incisions to spread, resulting in scars that are large and noticeable. This is particularly a problem for alopecia reductions and flaps because the scars are usually located in visible areas of the scalp.

You can gently shampoo your scalp the day after the procedure and every day after that. If you want to use hairspray, it must be washed off daily. While shampooing, make sure the water is a gentle spray rather than a strong stream that hits the incisions. Be sure to follow all of your physician's instructions.

Three days after surgery, to help remove the crusting around suture lines, it may be helpful to soak the area in warm water for five to ten minutes prior to washing. You can accomplish this by sitting in the tub and letting the back of your scalp sink below the surface level of the water. Never rub the scabs with a towel, rather pat your head dry. Be especially careful when combing hair that may be trapped in the scabs. Do not force the comb!

Taking vitamins after surgery is fine. We recommend taking 800 IU of vitamin E daily starting forty-eight hours after surgery and continuing for at least one month. Vitamin C can be taken at 2000 milligrams a day, starting the week prior to surgery and continuing for one month. If you are already taking multi-vitamins and/or other herbal supplements, check with your doctor to find out which ones you can safely take during and after the procedure.

Post-Operative Swelling

The cause of post-operative swelling is not completely understood, but is believed to be caused by an interruption of the scalp's lymphatic drainage system and inflammation from the surgery. About three days after surgery, swelling may begin in the forehead and extend to the area around the eyes. There seems to be a relationship between the presence of swelling and the number of grafts placed, the number of previous surgeries done, and the area of the head being worked on.

To help prevent swelling, apply an ice pack or cold compress to the forehead and temples for fifteen minutes at a time, several times a day, starting the day after surgery—regardless of whether any swelling is visible or not. Never place the ice pack directly on the grafts. Also, sleeping with your head elevated for several nights after surgery helps contain swelling. Use multiple pillows to prop up your back and head, or try sleeping in a recliner. If swelling appears (even after taking these preventive measures), it will usually decrease twenty-four hours after it began. The patient can try "milking" the forehead area by gently pressing the fluid away from the eyes towards the temples as soon as swelling begins. This may also help prevent black eyes.

Physical Activity

Vigorous exercise causes a rise in blood pressure and increased perspiration; it may also cause accidental bumps and bruising to the head, which, in turn, may lead to infection, bleeding from the wounds, or graft dislodgment. You must, therefore, suspend all forms of such activity for seven to ten days after surgery. This includes participation in sports such as tennis, jogging, racquetball, swimming, and biking. Weightlifting or any work that involves pushing, pulling, or lifting heavy objects is equally discouraged.

Potential Complications After Surgery

Any surgery can have possible post-operative complications. Among hair-rearrangements, transplantation has the lowest percentage of these problems. Flaps and reductions have a higher percentage because of their invasive natures. The most common complications include infection, bleeding, numbness, itching, graft elevation or depression, graft compression, keloids, ateriovenous fistulas, and improper wound healing.

- **Infection.** The most common signs of infection at the site of grafts or incisions include pain, redness, swelling, heat, and discharge. Swelling caused by infection is different from the general post-operative swelling that sometimes occurs after surgery. It tends to remain localized in the affected area, which is typically hot, tender, and accompanied by a discharge. Contact your doctor at the first sign of any of these symptoms. When treated with antibiotics, an infection can be contained quickly and rarely affects hair growth. Those who take antibiotics before and after the surgery as a preventive measure rarely, if ever, develop an infection.

- **Bleeding.** The most common cause of post-op bleeding after hair surgery is from an accidental knock or blow to the head. If this occurs, apply direct pressure to the site for ten to fifteen minutes. If the area continues to bleed, call your doctor immediately. And if a graft is knocked out from a trauma (even combing) to the head, don't hesitate calling the doctor.

- **Numbness.** Many fine nerve endings are cut during hair rearrangement, resulting in decreased sensitivity or numbness along and around surgical wounds, especially those in the donor area. This is a temporary condition. The nerves will reconnect over a period of one to four months, but can take as long as eighteen months to fully heal. Instead of numbness, some patients experience just the opposite, feeling pain and heightened sensitivity in areas of the scalp. This occurs because the nerves are adjusting to their new connections.

- **Itching.** Itching is a sign of healing, and as grafts and incisions begin to heal, itching typically occurs near the surgical wounds. Do not scratch! Instead, apply a topical antibiotic and/or cortisone cream to the area for relief.

- **Graft elevation and depression.** Although rare, grafts that don't heal evenly with the scalp, but are either raised or depressed, can occur as a result of mini/micrografting. Called *cobblestoning,* unevenly healed grafts are the result of poor transplanting techniques. In some cases, the grafts will alter their positions, usually within a year, and become flush with the surface of the scalp. Leveling the areas through dermabrasion or by shaving the raised skin with scalpels are other options.

- **Graft compression.** This complication can occur when larger grafts that contain many follicular units are placed into a site, and, due to the nature of healing, the connective tissue fibers in the skin compress the grafts, causing them to lie close to one another. The resulting appearance resembles a "bundle" or "rope" of hair emerging from a single graft site. One way to correct this problem is through graft removal. Another solution is to camouflage the compression by grafting follicular units into the surrounding areas.

- **Keloids.** Unusually large raised scars, keloids most commonly occur in Blacks. Any history of unusual healing should be brought to your surgeon's attention. Before undergoing surgery, a trial graft can be planted to observe how your body heals.

- **Arteriovenous fistulas.** Usually occurring in the donor area, arteriovenous fistulas are small blood-filled sacs that form when a vein heals to a nearby artery. They feel like small balloons beneath the skin. Contact your doctor immediately if you suspect that you have a fistula. Based on its proximity to the skin's surface, a fistula can be removed surgically, or left to resolve on its own, which usually occurs within eighteen months.

- **Improper wound healing.** An incision or other surgical wound that opens during the healing process is an indication of poor surgical technique. This happens most commonly with alopecia reductions. It results when too much skin has been removed and there is too much tension on the remaining skin, which is closed with sutures or staples.

The Future Schedule

The scheduling of future surgeries depends on the technique you have chosen. If you have undergone an FUT, no future schedule is necessary—at least not immediately. Because of the nature of this type of transplant, you may decide that you are completely happy with the density of your hair and the change in your appearance after only one surgical session.

If you elect to have another follicular unit or micrograft surgery, typically you should wait eight to ten months. This allows complete healing and full growth of the transplanted hair. A surgery performed before the grafts of a prior session have had sufficient time to grow has the potential to damage the earlier transplants. This is because micrografts and follicular units leave no visible evidence of their location, that is, until the hair actually begins to grow. Therefore, a surgeon may inadvertently make an incision at the same location of a previous graft and damage the follicle before it has had an opportunity to grow.

If you have had an alopecia reduction, flap, or mini/micrografts, you will need further surgeries to make your hair appear natural and undetectable. Usually, a second reduction or minigraft transplant procedure can be planned as early as six to eight weeks following the previous surgery.

BOGUS SURGICAL PROCEDURES

Several procedures exist in the field of hair transplantation that are bogus—plain and simple. They are ineffective and some are potentially harmful. Currently, the most prevalent of these treatments is the use of lasers, although implants and arterial ligations are also being performed throughout the world. We discuss these procedures briefly to make you aware of their existence and to warn you about them.

Lasers

Lasers, which are used in place of scalpels to create recipient sites, have been embraced by a small portion of the hair-rearrangement community. Most surgeons agree that the laser's place within this field is merely a research instrument at this time. Sadly, it is being used as a marketing tool to lure potential patients who are susceptible to the hype that is associated with laser technology.

Many leading doctors who have been investigating lasers for use in hair transplantation acknowledge several problems. As with any incision made in the skin, lasers leave scars. Lasers can also cause thermal (heat) damage to the scalp, impeding hair growth and causing color change in the scalp. When using lasers, there is little room for error, making their use especially dangerous in untrained hands. Moreover, the initial purchase and maintenance of the laser machine is costly, and those costs are passed onto the patient.

The use of lasers might be valuable to aid the transplantation process at some point in the future. Currently, however, their use is fairly ineffective—capable of causing more harm than good.

Arterial Ligation

Arterial ligation involves tying off either or both of the temporal arteries that supply blood to the top of the head. The reasoning behind this procedure is that if blood cannot get to the top of the head, the hormones that trigger baldness cannot interact with the hair follicles. If it were indeed possible to stop all blood flow to the top of the scalp, eventually your entire scalp would die and fall off—which would certainly stop the balding process. More important, though, tying off the temporal arteries cannot stop the flow of blood to the top of the scalp because they do not supply all of the blood to the area. All of the arteries to the scalp are connected like a spider web. This means that any main artery can supply blood to all points. Don't even entertain this option. In addition to being risky, it simply doesn't work!

Synthetic Implants

Synthetic implants are fibers that are shaped into hair-like strands, and then implanted directly in the scalp as if they were real hair. Using these implants means that grafts are not needed from the donor area. In addition to the implants being difficult to maintain, this technique has other serious drawbacks. Because these hairs are foreign bodies, their presence in the scalp typically results in severe swelling and redness, and almost always leads to serious infection. Although, thankfully, this procedure is now illegal in the United States, it is a flourishing practice in countries like Japan, Australia, and Italy.

CONCLUSION

Although alopecia reductions and skin flaps are possible options for treating male pattern baldness, modern hair-transplantation techniques lead the race as better choices. Among their many positive features, properly performed hair transplants can provide good coverage, excellent density, and a natural appearance.

The potential for the success of any surgical procedure, however, is often matched with an equal potential for failure and damage. Chapter 7 explores the reconstruction techniques that are used to repair the mistakes made by earlier cosmetic surgery, as well as damage to the head and face caused by accident or disease.

7

Repair and Reconstruction

"We do it right, 'cause we do it twice."

—*ANONYMOUS*

Ever since doctors began performing cosmetic surgery on the face and head, there have also been problems and complications caused by these procedures that affect both appearance and hair growth. In some instances, instead of improving the way a person looks, these procedures can create new problems or make existing ones worse. Most of these complications are the result of either faulty technique or inexperience on the part of the surgeon. Perhaps the doctor did not properly estimate the patient's final balding pattern or understand the aesthetic rules of hairline placement.

In addition to those who have undergone surgery for cosmetic reasons, victims of accidents, trauma, or disease may also need repair or reconstructive surgery. Fortunately, there is much that can be done.

This chapter begins with an exploration of some of the common problems and various cosmetic needs involved with hair restoration, and then presents the most appropriate solutions available. Following this discussion, a special section addresses the problems that are most likely to affect women—although men may find much of the information in this section useful as well. Finally, the costs that are involved in these repair and reconstruction techniques are presented.

A UNIQUE FIELD

Surgical repair and reconstruction of the head, face, and neck straddle the fields of reconstructive plastic surgery and head and neck surgery. The specific techniques used for repairing problems that are related to hair rearrangement are not taught in most medical programs. Often, it is only the correct placement of hair that can complete a cosmetic repair on the head or face. Currently, only a small percentage of surgeons who specialize in hair rearrangement have also had training in reconstructive surgery.

While more and better options are available than ever before, surgical repair can still be a difficult process at best. In many cases, the patient does not have adequate donor reserves to cover all of the bald areas. Therefore, the planning of repair work is especially critical because not a hair can be wasted. To plan correctly and to achieve a normal appearance, the doctor must be experienced in proper hair-transplantation technique and design, as well as repair and reconstruction—this point cannot be overstated.

Because of the high visibility of the head and face, cosmetic problems in this area are often more upsetting than those on other parts of the body. When determining the best course of action, the surgeon must consider a number of factors. The reconstruction must make aesthetic sense and also conserve donor hair. Attention to the hairline and forelock is absolutely paramount. Because the frontal hairline is the most visible part of the reconstruction, all resources must first be used to fix it in order to achieve a normal appearance. Once this part of the head has been addressed, other areas can be assessed for repair.

PROBLEMS AND SOLUTIONS

Most cosmetic problems resulting from improper hair surgery, accident, or disease fall into one of three categories—inappropriate hairlines, plugginess, and scars. Other problems also exist, such as slot deformations caused by alopecia reductions and facial hair abnormalities involving sideburns, beards, and moustaches. A variety of solutions are available, including follicular unit transplantation, tissue expansion, pruning grafts, and poaching of the donor area.

Improper Hairlines

If a person has an unnatural frontal hairline, the surgeon should always start the reconstruction there. When improperly placed, poorly shaped, pluggy, or abrupt, a hairline will appear unnatural and detectable. Often these problems overlap.

Just as in real estate, when it comes to hair rearrangement, location plays a critical role. As explained in Chapter 6, the correct hairline should be designed according to the rule of thirds, which governs the aesthetic proportions of the face and head. Once again, the distance from the hairline to the eyebrow should measure the same distance as that from the eyebrow to the bottom of the nose, or from the bottom of the nose to the chin. The goal when placing a hairline is to have it provide balance and a frame for the face.

An inappropriately high hairline is easiest to fix. The correct hairline is simply drawn below the existing one, and then the area is filled in with grafts. Grafts are also added to thicken the "former" hairline, which has become part of the interior forelock area.

The term "improperly shaped" hairline often refers to those that are concave in shape, indenting inward toward the top of the head, as seen in Figure 7.1 below. After drawing the properly shaped hairline, incorporating as much hair as possible from the existing hairline, the surgeon will then fill in any bald spaces with follicular unit transplants.

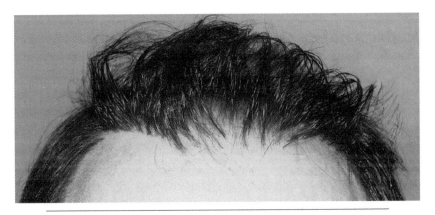

FIGURE 7.1. CONCAVE HAIRLINE
In this example of an improperly constructed hairline,
the patient's frontal hairline is concave in shape.

Lacking a soft transition from the forehead, this unnaturally abrupt hairline resembles a "wall of hair."

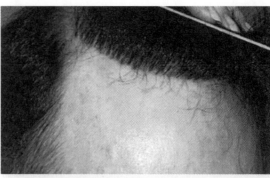

In one session, 600 follicular units were added to create a softer, more natural look.

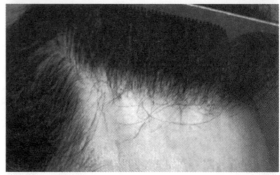

FIGURE 7.2. ABRUPT HAIRLINE

An abrupt hairline is one that has no gradual transition from the hairless forehead to the frontal hairline. It typically looks like a "wall" of hair. Figure 7.2 above shows an abrupt hairline that was softened with the placement of follicular unit grafts. Often, multiple sessions are required to remedy this problem.

A more serious and difficult hairline problem to correct is the one that is too low and too wide. Obviously, additional grafts are not the answer, as they would only make this problem worse. Instead, the hairline must be raised and reshaped to be age appropriate. Several techniques can aid in this process. After drawing a line indicating where the hairline should go to appear most natural looking, the surgeon can correct the problem by removing any and all extraneous hair. In most cases, the hair that is removed can be transplanted into other areas.

Another technique used to fix a low hairline is the *triangle wedge resection*, as seen in Figure 7.3 on the facing page. This procedure is like a small alopecia reduction in which unwanted hair-bearing skin above the temples is removed to create a proper shape. The resulting wound is then covered with hairless skin that has been stretched from the forehead area. The resulting scar can then be camouflaged with follicular unit grafts.

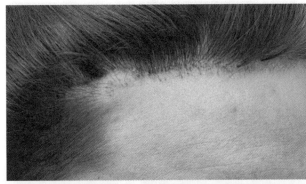

This patient's hairline was placed too low in the temple area.

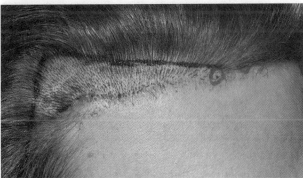

The surgeon marked the area that was to be removed, trimmed the hair, and performed a triangle wedge resection—skin from the forehead was stretched to cover the wound.

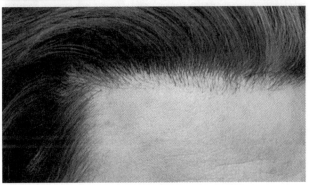

The shape of a normal hairline was restored.

Photos courtesy of Dr. Michael Beehner, Saratoga Springs, New York.

7.3. TRIANGLE WEDGE RESECTION

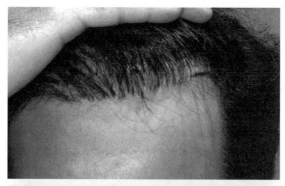

Poor transplantation surgery resulted in this patient's pluggy frontal hairline.

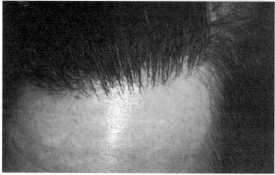

During the repair, which was performed in two sessions, approximately 1,500 follicular unit grafts were placed.

FIGURE 7.4. PLUGGY HAIRLINE

Another hairline that requires repair is the one that is pluggy in appearance, as seen in Figure 7.4 above. Usually the result of an unfinished or an improperly planned transplant, a pluggy hairline has a tufted or corn row appearance instead of a natural growth pattern. Often the remedy is no more complicated than simply adding more grafts of the same size until the plugginess is eliminated. Follicular unit transplants can then be added to create a natural-looking softness zone.

Plugginess

Plugginess can exist anywhere in the transplanted hair, not just at the hairline. The most common way to correct plugginess is by transplanting more hair into the affected area until the pluggy look is eliminated.

But where do these grafts come from? For those with enough

donor hair, the answer is obvious. But what about those who have been told that their donor area is used up due to prior graft harvestings? For them, a technique called *poaching* is a possible solution. Poaching involves going into a seemingly used-up donor area and removing a strip of skin that contains hair and as many old scars as possible. By using the FUT technique of graft preparation, completely viable follicular units can be excised from the scarred tissue and then transplanted. As an added bonus, the surgeon can often consolidate multiple scars into one.

Be aware that plugginess is not as simple to correct when it is compounded by graft compression. As discussed in Chapter 6, compression occurs when larger grafts containing several follicular units are placed into a site and the connective tissue compresses them together. The result looks much like a thick bundle of hair growing out of the scalp, as seen in Figure 7.5 below. This occurs

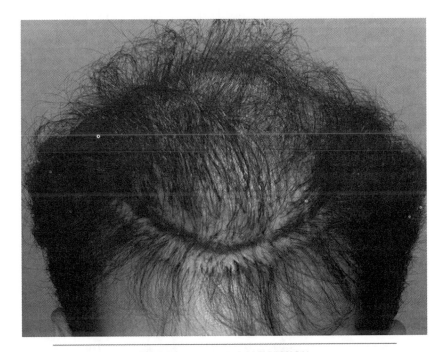

FIGURE 7.5. GRAFT COMPRESSION

The plugginess of this poorly performed transplant is compounded by graft compression, which looks like a rope of hair. Graft compression results when large grafts containing too many follicles are placed into a site, and then become pressed together as the surrounding connective tissue heals.

most often in dark-haired patients. A pluggy look is accentuated when compression is present. In such cases, the doctor must make a judgement call to either remove or thin the compressed grafts, or continue transplanting additional smaller grafts to help camouflage the plugginess.

A surgeon may also consider *pruning*. This technique involves removing the compressed grafts completely if they are small, or partially if they are large. The removed or "pruned" grafts can then be dissected under a microscope and replanted as follicular units, since useable hair should never be thrown away.

Scars

Scars, which are typically caused by prior surgery, accident, or disease, are serious cosmetic problems anywhere on the head. Tissue expansion and scar revisions are the most common solutions for visible scars. Occasionally, hair transplants can also be used to help cover them.

Poorly performed alopecia reductions often leave scars on bald areas that may be wide, depressed, or elevated. Adding to their visibility is the fact that scars are characteristically lighter in color than the surrounding skin. If the scar was caused by a prior surgery, a *scar revision* is usually the first step. This technique involves surgically removing the old scar, and then closing up the wound with as little tension as possible. Although this will not eliminate the scar completely, it should result in one that is finer and less visible than the original one. No ethical surgeon will ever tell you that he can guarantee an undetectable scar.

Scars along the frontal hairline that are caused by flap surgery are also problematic. Even though the scar may be located against the hair of the flap, it is usually visible and difficult to conceal. Normally, the transition from bald forehead to hairy forelock is gradual; however, a flap causes this transition to be abrupt, making the scar noticeable. The same problem occurs with *circumferential scars,* which run along the top border of the fringe and are caused by extensive scalp lifts.

The seemingly logical solution to flap and circumferential scars is to simply transplant hair into them. For flap scars, this can be a successful option, as the hair in a properly performed flap will remain stable, however, this is not the case for most circumferential scars. If the individual continues to lose hair, a long ribbon of bald scalp will appear as the fringe recedes from the scar that has been covered with transplants. Then the surgeon must transplant thousands of hairs into this bald strip, which is not the best use of the finite donor reserve. Circumferential scars are, therefore, best left alone.

Individuals with large areas of damaged scalp due to burns, lacerations, tumors, or radiation treatment can benefit greatly from scar revision. Depending on where the scar or damage is located, the use of tissue expansion can sometimes aid in the complete removal of the scar or damaged area. Tissue expansion (discussed in detail in Chapter 6) involves stretching hair-bearing areas of the scalp, which are then lifted up to better cover bald areas. For cases in which the scalp is scarred or damaged, an expansion can help stretch the hair-bearing skin to cover these areas. Keep in mind, however, that qualifying for this procedure depends on overall scalp looseness. Some individuals may be "stretched out" due to a previous surgery involving tissue expansion or an alopecia reduction. Once the scar tissue from a revision or a removal has been reduced to a minimum and an adequate blood supply is re-established, hair grafts can be placed. Of course, the number of available grafts will always depend on the hair density of the donor area.

Slot Deformation and White Sidewalls

As explained in Chapter 6, a *slot deformation* is caused by alopecia reduction surgery in which the opposing fringes are brought together at the top of the head. This causes abnormal hair direction, and usually a visible scar that runs along the length of the head where the fringes have been joined.

Attempted solutions for slot deformation problems are among the least successful types of repairs. One possible solution is a scar revision to make the smallest scar possible. If the individual is lucky, he will have plenty of donor hair that can be transplanted into the frontal zone for better coverage. And it would be even better if the hair is coarse and curly—characteristics that lend themselves to improved density. Another possible solution is the *three hair-bearing flaps transposition.* Created by Patrick Frechet, MD, of France, this procedure is specifically designed to correct slot deformations and re-establish normal hair direction. Three skin flaps are cut and placed in a way to give the hair proper direction. However, if the individual continues to bald after this procedure, more scars will become visible across the back of the head.

White sidewalls describe unnaturally wide hairless areas that are located along the nape of the neck and around the ears. They are caused by a raised hairline—often the result of extensive scalp lifting, performed during alopecia reductions. There are two possible surgical solutions for this problem. One procedure involves transplanting hair into the area; however, this wastes precious grafts that can be better used in the front area of the head. The other solution is to stretch the skin through tissue expansion and then lower the hairline back towards the ear. Unfortunately, because of the original alopecia reduction, which caused the sidewalls to begin with, the person's scalp may already be stretched out. In such a case, tissue expansion is not possible. The only remaining option is to simply let the hair grow so that it's long enough to cover the area.

Beard and Mustache Reconstruction

Follicular unit transplantation has made beard and mustache reconstruction viable. Men with naturally scant or light beards who desire better coverage, or those whose beards have been damaged by accident or disease, can have follicular unit grafts placed in the area. In addition to scalp hair, hair that is taken from under the chin can also be used for transplantation. Moderation is the key when reconstructing a beard or mustache, which can require a lot of hair. Since the donor supply is finite and may not be enough to cover both the beard and the bald areas of the head, the physician must use discretion.

REPAIRS FOR WOMEN

In addition to the repair of problems resulting from unnatural hairlines and improper grafting, which involves the same techniques used on men, some women require reconstruction of frontal and temporal hairlines after having facial plastic surgery. This includes repairing scars and replacing damaged sideburns and temple hair. Women may also need to repair damaged eyebrows and eyelashes caused by disease or trauma.

Scars from Cosmetic Surgery

For women, problems with scarring most often occur after some type of cosmetic surgery involving the face—usually browlifts and facelifts.

For cosmetic *browlifts,* an incision is usually made behind the frontal hairline, and the entire forehead is elevated in an effort to raise the eyebrows. Then the excess hair-bearing skin is removed and the wound is sewn shut. The incision is made behind the hairline to camouflage the scar, which may still be visible in some cases. Surgeons who want to avoid raising the hairline too much may make the incision for the browlift in front of the hairline. Of course, the scar will then be visible.

The first step in correcting these problems is always to evaluate the scar. No hair transplantation should be done until both the plastic surgeon and the transplant surgeon agree that the scar cannot be made any finer or thinner through a scar revision. Also keep in mind that a revision may also be the most economical way to begin the reconstruction process because it can reduce the number of grafts needed to cover the scar. If a revision is necessary, the patient should return to the surgeon who performed the original procedure. Most surgeons will do the follow-up surgery free of charge or for a minimal fee. Of course, it's always best to discuss these charges for possible scar revision *prior* to the initial surgery. Once the scar has been revised, follicular unit transplantation techniques can be used to lower an elevated hairline, or to transplant hair into any visible scar along the frontal hairline.

Incisions for *facelifts* are often made in the temporal hair along the front of the ears and under the earlobes. They continue behind the ears and into the hair. After the skin is trimmed and resewn, two problems can arise. First, scarring may be clearly noticeable in the temple areas and behind the ears as seen in Figure 7.6 on page 142, especially if the hair is pulled up into a ponytail. Second, sideburns may be completely lost as a result of the facelift, as shown

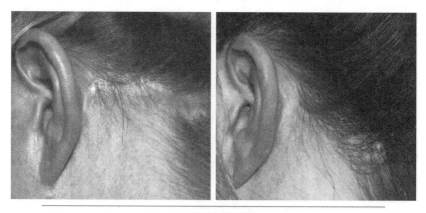

7.6. SCAR REPAIR
The scarring behind this woman's ear is a complication from facelift surgery.
In one session, 225 follicular unit grafts were placed to hide the scar.

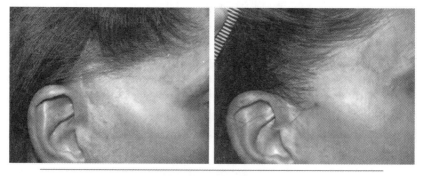

7.7. SIDEBURN RECONSTRUCTION
Loss of sideburns and scarring above the ear often follows facelift surgery.
In this case, coverage was achieved with 511 follicular unit grafts,
which were placed in a single session.

in Figure 7.7 above. This complication is actually pretty common, and one that women should discuss with their plastic surgeons prior to surgery. This way, arrangements can be made for a hair-replacement surgeon who is competent in sideburn reconstruction.

Elevated Hairlines

An abnormally high hairline can be the result of a surgical proce-dure, particularly a browlift. It can also be a variation of normal female hair growth. Elevated hairlines tend to be hereditary—

mom and grandma often have the same one. Most women with high hairlines find that wearing bangs is a good option. However, there are some women whose hairlines are simply too high for bangs, which won't lie naturally.

For the woman who is bothered by a high hairline, follicular unit transplantation is a good option for lowering it. Of course, the extent of how far down the forehead one can go with transplants depends on the amount of available donor hair. Another consideration is proper aesthetic placement. As discussed in Chapter 6, women typically have different, more intricately shaped frontal hairlines than men, requiring intensive thought and planning prior to transplantation. To achieve hair density that matches the density found on the top of the head, multiple surgeries are often necessary. For this reason, time and cost factors should be considered.

Another option for correcting this problem is stretching the scalp through tissue expansion and then lowering the hairline. In most cases, this allows the surgeon to advance the hairline as far as needed, and the results are faster than they are through grafting. Keep in mind that having an expander in place for several weeks will cause an abnormal appearance; however, existing hair can usually be styled to hide it.

Eyebrow and Eyelash Reconstruction

Bald areas of the eyebrow can result from excessive tweezing, hypothyroidism, trichotillomania, and naturally poor density. A growing number of individuals who have had their eyebrows pierced and then decorated with rings and studs may be left with bald spots there as well.

It is important to note that if medical treatment is indicated, it should always precede any cosmetic surgical procedure for men or women. For example, treating hypothyroidism with the appropriate medication may cause the regrowth of some hair. Therefore, the area shouldn't be evaluated for surgical treatment until the medical therapy has been completed. In the case of trichotillomania—a condition in which the individual is constantly plucking out hair—no surgical reconstruction should begin until the underlying psychological condition has been treated.

Even more than with the female hairline, proper eyebrow

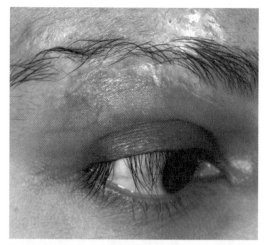

Trauma caused the loss of hair and scarring to this eyebrow.

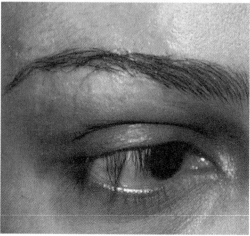

After one session in which 52 single follicular unit grafts were placed, a normal eyebrow contour was established.

7.8. EYEBROW RECONSTRUCTION

reconstruction requires great attention to detail. Single hair follicular units should be used to achieve the most natural-looking eyebrows, as seen in Figure 7.8 above. And since the transplanted hair came from the head, it will continue to grow in the eyebrow area, requiring occasional trimming.

Loss of eyelashes can be the result of trichotillomania or a damaged eyelid. Unfortunately, eyelash reconstruction can be very problematic. Eyelash hair is very fine and genetically programmed to curl away from the opening of the eye. Scalp hairs tend to grow straight, and once transplanted, can grow directly into the eye. This may lead to *trichiasis*—an irritating complication that can result in corneal damage. In this situation, the offending hair must be removed immediately.

COST

Costs for cosmetic repair and reconstruction for hair loss are very similar to those outlined in Chapter 6 for the original procedures. This is because the same surgeries are being performed in slightly different ways. Follicular unit transplantation techniques range from $3.00 to $12.00 per graft for any area of the head or face. The cost of an alopecia reduction ranges from $3,000 to $5,500. When tissue expansion is also part of the reduction, the cost nearly doubles.

CONCLUSION

The modern techniques of tissue expansion and follicular unit transplantation offer options for repair and reconstruction that weren't even a consideration in the recent past. Even with such advancements, guaranteed solutions are not possible for everyone. However, for many individuals, these techniques can lead to significantly improved appearance.

PART III

The Right Decision

8.

Decisions, Decisions

"What he hath scanted men in hair,
he hath given them in wit."

—WILLIAM SHAKESPEARE, *COMEDY OF ERRORS*

The previous chapters have provided a wealth of valuable information on the available options for hair replacement. But after all is said and done, it is *you* who must make the decision on the best course of action. Are you going to accept your hair loss, or will you attempt to replace it? And if your decision is the latter, which option seems best for you? A hair addition? A surgical procedure? A pharmaceutical therapy?

By examining a number of important issues, such as time considerations, cost factors, and personal preferences, and by reviewing the pros and cons of each hair-replacement method, this chapter is designed to aid you in your decision. It will help you focus on your personal needs and goals, so you can decide on the best means of achieving them. Just keep in mind that these guidelines are meant only to shed light on the various options. You will still need the guidance and expertise of a qualified hair-replacement professional to confirm that the treatment you are considering can work in your particular case.

ESTABLISHING YOUR GOALS

Before jumping into the fray, always take the time to consider your ultimate goal. Most people who pick up this book have already decided to do something about their hair loss. Whether you are one of these people or if you are still examining all of your options, now is a good time to remind yourself that getting hair replacement in any form is a choice—your choice. No one should force you into any decision. Be sure to take whatever time you need to review your goals slowly, calmly, and rationally.

Clearly, many individuals choose to live with their hair loss, and there are many positive aspects of this decision. First, you will always look normal and natural. Second, there is no chance of disfigurement or even disappointment in the outcome of a procedure. And of course, let's not forget about the financial advantage—you'll avoid the many costs involved. This is also a decision that enables you to change your mind in the future. Once you've committed to surgery, there's no going back.

Be aware that although you will probably always care about the way you look, your definition of baldness will change over time. To a thirty-year-old man, baldness can mean a loss of hair that occurs anywhere on his head—front, top, or back. To a sixty-year-old, it means having no hair on the front half of his head. Why such a difference in the points of view? It has to do with a change in the person's frame of reference. When a balding thirty-year-old looks at his peer group, he is likely to be in the minority with his hair loss. By contrast, when a man is in his sixties, nearly 70 percent of his peers will be either bald or experiencing thinning on the back of their heads, so he won't feel so alone with his condition. However, a high percentage of men in that age group will still have hair on the front half of their heads. This area then becomes the standard for his definition of "baldness." What you want today may not be what you will want ten years from now.

Of course, the alternative to accepting hair loss is opting for some form of replacement. If you know that this is what you want but aren't sure which option will serve you best, taking a realistic look at a number of important issues will help in your decision.

REVIEWING THE ISSUES

Once you have decided that you want hair, you must honestly assess exactly how much you want, and exactly what you will and will not do to restore it. Those experiencing hair loss have different priorities and, therefore, different boundaries. When it comes to cost, some men will spare no expense, while others may have to adhere to a clear and well-planned budget. Some individuals will be willing to devote lots of time to the particular process involved, while others won't be agreeable to such a sacrifice. Still other issues, such as age and the extent and type of hair loss, may also come into play. It is only by examining each and every issue and assessing how they affect your situation and personal preferences that you will be able to make a decision that's right for you.

As you consider the following options, you may find that an answer to one question will change upon answering another. Be flexible; but most of all, be sure that you are honest with yourself. There is no right or wrong answer—there's only the one that makes you comfortable.

Age

When it comes to surgical procedures and pharmaceutical options, age can be a factor. In the vast majority of cases, younger men—those under age twenty-five—have only limited hair loss due to male pattern baldness. Only the most conservative approaches, if any, should be used in these cases. Unless the extent or likely progression of hair loss is evident, men in this age group are rarely candidates for surgery. Generally speaking, the older a person is, the better the candidate for transplantation. The balding pattern is likely to be evident, allowing the surgeon to properly plan for the particular procedure. As a result, the recipient is more likely to achieve positive results from surgery. Age is not much of a factor for women, even though their natural hair-loss patterns can be progressive. Whether or not a woman is a good candidate depends more on the characteristics of her donor hair, not her age.

When it comes to repairing damage caused by trauma or accident, age is not necessarily a factor for surgery. However, prior to any procedure, the future hair loss that is likely to occur due to male pattern baldness must be considered. This is important for all candidates, particularly younger men. Because they can be used by men of any age, hair additions can be an excellent choice for coverage under these circumstances.

Pharmaceuticals, like Rogaine (or other minoxidil products) and Propecia, can be used by males over the age of eighteen. In general, these medications, which seem to be more effective at preserving existing hair than growing new ones, are most beneficial for younger men who are in the early stages of hair loss. As discussed in Chapter 5, there is a greater chance that these individuals will have more vellus or intermediate hairs, which react best to these medications.

Before a woman begins pharmaceutical treatment for hair loss, she must be certain that it is the result of female pattern baldness, not an underlying medical condition. Once this has been confirmed through a medical examination, a woman can consider treatment with minoxidil. Propecia is not indicated for women.

Cause and Extent of Hair Loss

Regardless of the amount of hair loss or its cause, a cosmetic hair addition is always a viable option. In fact, for certain conditions like alopecia totalis, which cannot be treated surgically or pharmaceutically, hair additions are the only option.

As mentioned earlier, the best candidates for Rogaine and Propecia are those whose pattern baldness is in a mild to moderate stage. Because these drugs are most effective at preserving existing hair, typically, they have little effect on those who have extensive hair loss.

With the exception of alopecia areata, alopecia totalis, and scarring alopecias, surgery can effectively treat most types of hair loss. Because alopecia areata affects the area of the scalp where the baldness is occurring, the transplants may not "take." Scarring alopecias, which may affect the recipient area much like alopecia areata, may also prevent new grafts from growing. Those with alopecia totalis experience hair loss over the entire scalp, which means there is no "donor area" from which to take grafts.

Desired Coverage

How much hair do you want? Are you willing to compromise on this issue? These are vitally important questions. Many individuals will say they want all of their hair back, but realistically, the response should be based on one's age. Younger men tend to want full or nearly full coverage, while older men, who have lived longer with their hair loss and are more used to it, tend to be less demanding.

No matter what your age, if you desire to have every inch of your scalp covered with hair, a hair addition is your best bet. Regardless of the amount of hair loss and when it occurs, only a hair addition can provide complete coverage safely and permanently. If you can accept compromise—trading coverage or density for complete undetectability—then surgery can be a good option for you. Some men feel that hair additions don't look natural enough and want only their own hair. Only surgery can satisfy this need.

If you cannot decide how much hair you want or what compromises you are willing to make, don't commit to any procedure. You might, however, consider pharmaceutical options if you are a good candidate for them. They can be a good way to get the ball rolling while giving yourself time to make a decision.

Time and Maintenance

Time is another important factor—it takes into consideration both the time needed to get your new hair, whether natural or synthetic, as well as the time necessary for maintaining it. How long are you willing to wait to get your new hair? How much time are you willing to spend in the offices of doctors or other hair-care providers? Once you have your hair, how much time are you willing or able to spend maintaining it?

If you decide to get a hair addition, don't expect it to be ready overnight. An addition requires several appointments to determine its initial design and then subsequent fittings once it is ready. Depending on their shape, color, and size, most additions take about six to eight weeks to be manufactured, although a custom order can take over three months.

All hair additions require maintenance on a regular basis. The amount of time this entails will vary depending on the type. As discussed in Chapter 4, some removable additions need to be maintained daily, while others may require attention every two weeks or so. Both permanent and removable additions call for regular cleaning, occasional tightening, and intermittent repairs, including the replacement of damaged hairs. In spite of all the time involved with the preparation and upkeep of a hair addition (which may or may not be of concern to you) once you put it on, the change in your appearance is immediate.

Surgery, on the other hand, is more time-consuming—at least initially. Transplantation requires surgery, usually an entire day. Recovery time for follicular unit transplants (FUT) is usually four to seven days, and up to two weeks for mini/micrografting. Some of the transplanted hairs should begin growing after two months, and by ten months, most of the hairs will have grown. Depending on the amount of hair density you want, multiple sessions may be required. With FUT, you may need at least two sessions, which should be spaced nine to ten months apart. Mini/micrografting techniques take longer than FUT to achieve the density, undetectability, and hair length you may desire. This process may take several years to complete because of the number of sessions required.

Of course, once you have your new hair, it will be *your* hair—not a cosmetic addition—and you will not have to schedule any additional time, other than haircuts, to maintain it. Many people feel that the results are worth the wait and any possible aggravation. However, you are the one who must live through the process. Can you handle the emotional aspects of such disruption to your work and social life?

Pharmaceuticals can take anywhere from six to ten months to work. The results may come in the form of visible hair growth or a cessation of hair loss. This can be frustrating, especially since these medications require daily use and a recurring monthly expense. On one hand, Propecia, which involves only taking a pill, is relatively easy. Rogaine, on the other hand, must be applied twice a day to achieve possible results.

Cost Considerations

How much can you afford to spend on hair replacement? Cost is a major concern for many individuals. Obviously, costs will vary, but in the long run, hair additions and surgery usually end up costing similar amounts. The difference is *when* the money is spent.

When compared to transplantations, initially, hair additions cost less. A basic, well-made, well-designed removable addition can cost anywhere from $1,200 to $1,500. Depending on the type of attachment, the yearly maintenance costs can range from $600 for removable systems, to $3,000 for permanent types. Many people who wear removable additions also choose to clean them themselves. However, there are some services, such as replacing lost or broken hairs, that must be done by a qualified professional. Over the years, maintenance and replacement costs for an addition will add up, making them comparable to surgery.

Depending on the extent of hair loss and the total area involved in the procedure, transplantation surgery—from start to finish—averages $15,000 to $20,000. This is a sizeable amount of money to spend within a year or two; therefore, some doctors or hair clinics offer payment plans. In addition to the actual cost of the procedure, other expenses should be factored in, including the time taken off work for the surgery and healing time. Once again, the advantage of surgery is that once it's over, you're finished. You never have to do anything to your transplanted hair, because it's your own real hair. This is a powerful incentive to many men.

The cost of pharmaceutical therapies varies. Regular-strength Rogaine runs about $25 to $30 dollars a month; expect to pay another $5 to $10 for the extra-strength variety. The monthly cost of Propecia is around $40 to $50. Keep in mind that as increased numbers of medications for hair loss become available, the competition is likely to drive down their costs.

Personal Preferences

Your personal feelings and preferences regarding hair replacement should not be ignored. Men are especially sensitive to their likes and dislikes regarding their hair. For example, some men don't like the idea of wearing a hair addition because they feel it looks fake or doesn't feel secure on their heads. Others may feel squeamish at the thought of surgery, or simply reject the idea of any elective cosmetic procedure. Still others, fearing the possibility of side effects, may not want to take daily medication for several years.

Pay attention to your instincts and voice any concerns about the hair-replacement option in question. It is most helpful to talk with people who have already undergone the surgical procedure, are wearing the hair addition, or are using the medication you are considering. This is a good way to get a realistic perspective on the various options, which may help in your decision.

A QUICK SUMMARY

So far, this chapter has examined some major considerations when choosing a form of hair replacement. To further help in this important decision, the following discussions provide a brief summary of the pros and cons of each of the major options.

Cosmetic Hair Additions

Hair additions offer two obvious advantages over the other options. First, from the moment you put on an addition, there is an immediate change in your appearance. There's no waiting for implants to "take" or medications to begin working. Second, the health risks involved are minimal. Attachment methods pose the only potential problems, and include such minimal, short-termed side effects as minor skin irritations and allergic reactions. There are other favorable advantages to hair additions. Removable varieties offer a great deal of flexibility in choosing when and why to wear them. An addition is the only option that can promise complete coverage, including the crown area. Finally, most additions come with money-back guarantees.

Of course, hair additions also have their disadvantages. Many don't look natural, and maintenance is time-consuming. When someone gets a bad hair addition, it can be very embarrassing both to the wearer and his friends. Keep in mind, though, that bad hair additions usually look unnatural because they are either too dense, too dark in color, or the wrong size.

There are two categories of men for whom hair additions are an especially good option—those who are balding in their teens, and those who will not accept the limitations of surgery. For a seventeen-year-old boy, a hair addition is the only short-term answer, because surgery is never appropriate for anyone that young. And for those men who refuse to accept the compromises that are inherent in surgical treatment, such as the lengthy time of the process and coverage limitations, a hair addition is the perfect alternative. Women are often excellent candidates for hair additions.

Unlike men, they are more likely to feel comfortable wearing wigs, which are considered an acceptable fashion "accessory." Many women have worn them in the past either for fun or out of need.

Pharmaceutical Treatments

Pharmaceuticals have several positive aspects that make them perfectly viable choices for most individuals. First of all, the majority of men can experience a complete cessation or slowing of hair loss for several years when using Rogaine (or another minoxidil product) or Propecia. As warned in Chapter 5, Propecia is not indicated for women. Women can, however, get hair growth from using minoxidil alone. Another major advantage of these medications? Since they stimulate existing hair, the results are always natural looking. Any styling and/or maintenance problems tend to be minimal. Topically applied minoxidil, however, can leave the hair feeling sticky or dry.

If you are also considering surgery, it can be wise to try a pharmaceutical product first. The psychological value of exhausting every nonsurgical avenue before committing to surgery is enormous. We have heard this admission from a countless number of our patients. Another advantage of taking Propecia or minoxidil is that during the time it takes to see any possible results, you can be exploring other options. You may even decide to go natural and avoid hair replacement altogether.

Pharmaceutical products do not work for everyone. A significant number of men have found them to be ineffective. Furthermore, it can take up to six months to determine if the product is working or not. This means you may have to spend a substantial amount of both time and money before possibly discovering that the drug isn't working. Perhaps the greatest disadvantage of pharmaceuticals is that they cannot promise complete hair growth for anyone. The frontal zone of the head usually has a limited response to the therapy, if there is any at all. This area often requires another option to correct the hair loss.

Finally, because these therapies are more effective at preserving existing hair than growing new ones, they are most beneficial for younger men in the early stages of hair loss, not those with an advanced stage. In addition, anyone experiencing hair loss for any reason other than androgenetic alopecia should not use a pharmaceutical product.

Surgical Options

Hair-rearrangement surgery has many positive aspects. When done correctly, it is the best option for providing naturalness, undetectability, and good density. Furthermore, because your own hair is used, transplants allow for ease of styling and maintenance. When all of these factors are taken into consideration, surgery is often the best alternative to meet the patient's needs.

Of course, surgery is not without its disadvantages. First of all, no matter which procedure you choose, all are expensive. There are many good surgeons who perform mini/micrografts; however, if you are interested in a follicular unit transplant, finding a qualified surgeon may be difficult. Only a small, although growing, number of surgeons are qualified to perform FUTs effectively. (In the next chapter, we'll talk more about finding a qualified surgeon.) Many individuals find the time commitment required for transplantation surgery one of its biggest disadvantages. Although FUT has dramatically reduced the amount of time needed to get positive results, mini/micrografts require multiple sessions that span many months before completion.

Nevertheless, 99 percent of all balding and bald men, regardless of their degree of hair loss or their age, are perfectly acceptable candidates for hair transplantation. Of course, they must understand the supply/demand limitations imposed by their own balding patterns, and be willing to accept them.

CONCLUSION

At this point, you have received a wealth of information on all of the available hair-replacement choices. You may have already made the decision to pursue a certain option. The next chapter will further help by guiding you in your search for a competent, experienced, and honest hair-replacement provider.

9

The Savvy
Consumer

"Contrary to popular opinion, the hustle is not a new dance step—
it is an old business procedure."

—FRAN LEBOWITZ, AMERICAN WRITER

By the time you reach this chapter, you may have decided on a hair-restoration option. Your next step would be to find a qualified provider who can help you achieve your goal. This chapter is designed to help you in your search. Not only does it offer suggestions for locating possible providers, it also outlines important guidelines for helping in your assessment of them. It's important to zero in on the person who is both willing and capable of doing the best possible job for you. Rounding out the chapter is some solid advice to help you see through all of the hype that's out there—the special offers, the claims that seem too good to be true, the amazing but suspicious before-and-after photos, and more. You will have all the information, support, skills, and confidence you need to be a savvy consumer.

Always remember that whether you are buying a hair addition, using pharmaceuticals, or electing to have surgery, the decision you make is a major one and should be approached with care and concern. But keep in mind that this can also be an enjoyable process. Think about it. You are taking decisive action to change your appearance in a way that is going to bring you satisfaction, so try to be positive during your search. A good attitude will help you make wiser decisions. Just as important, don't rush to choose a provider—never settle. If someone makes you feel the least bit concerned or apprehensive, don't hesitate to continue your search until you find the person who has all of the qualities you want.

FINDING THE RIGHT PROVIDER

Don't expect to find the professional who is best-suited to fill your particular needs overnight. The process of getting names and recommendations is similar to a job search, requiring determination, stamina, and some good old-fashioned homework. So where does the journey begin? Depending on the replacement option you have chosen, there are lots of places to start looking—more than you might suspect.

No matter which avenue you are considering—surgery, cosmetic additions, or drugs—always try to start your search with a personal lead. If you know anyone who has had the procedure, uses the medication, or wears the type of addition you are interested in, begin your research there. (Of course, the person must be someone you feel comfortable in speaking with.) If you don't know anyone personally, try networking through friends, family members, and/or business associates, who may know someone you can contact. This way, you can see the work first-hand, and obtain some additional information about the provider *before* making contact.

Surgeons

More than with any other option, if you are considering a transplant, it's most helpful to connect with individuals who have already had the surgery. Transplantation, although considered minor surgery, is still an invasive procedure. Each session (of which there can be many) requires local anesthesia, a short healing period, and time spent waiting for the transplanted hair to grow. As seen in Chapter 6, depending on the type of transplant, the entire process can take over a year before completion. It is because of this major commitment of time, effort, and money that we strongly recommend seeing an example of the completed work first. Seeing and speaking with someone who has actually had the type of transplants you are considering will allow you to assess the quality of the work, determine if it meets your personal needs, and answer the critical question: *Would I want that procedure to be performed on me?* We also strongly recommend that you use a surgeon who performs these procedures exclusively.

In addition to getting leads from friends and family, consider contacting your family physician for referrals. Through their network of colleagues, many doctors are able to offer recommendations. And if you have undergone any cosmetic plastic surgery in the past or if you have a dermatologist, call them for recommendations. A simple phone call to a local medical or dermatology society may be beneficial as well. These societies are usually listed in the phone directory under the state, county, or city—for example, Los Angeles Medical Society or Colorado Dermatologic Society.

Remember, we strongly recommend that you go to a surgeon who performs hair-replacement surgeries exclusively. An excellent source for finding names of specialists in the field is The International Society of Hair Restoration Surgery (ISHRS)—the largest and most respected society in this field. It can provide a listing of members in good standing in your area. Keep in mind, however, that although a surgeon's name may be on the list, it does not imply anything about the quality of his or her work. By calling the doctor's office directly, you can learn if the surgeon performs a particular procedure. To contact the society, call 1-800-444-2737, or visit its website at www.ISHRS.org.

The Internet is another possible resource for finding surgeons in your area. Searching under "hair restoration" will turn up a number of websites that may offer leads for further investigation. We are familiar with three sites in particular that offer solid general information on hair restoration, as well as the names of highly qualified hair transplant surgeons. They are:

www.TheBaldTruth.com

www.HairTransplantNetwork.com

www.HairLossTalk.com

The doctors who are registered on these sites have been selected based upon an examination of their work and patient recommendations. They are listed by location, and any of their special qualifications are mentioned.

To further help in your search, we have provided a list of highly qualified surgeons in the Physician Referral List, beginning on page 189. These doctors were selected based on our personal knowledge of the outstanding quality of their work, as well as their good standing in the hair-replacement community. Although the names we have listed represent only a sampling of the many fine, highly skilled doctors available, we offer them as a possible starting point for your investigation.

A woman's search for a surgeon is more challenging, simply because the diagnosis of female pattern baldness is more difficult than that of male pattern baldness. It's important to find a doctor who has had a great deal of experience and interest in handling women's hair loss. Word of mouth or personal referrals from a family physician are the best avenues for obtaining contact names, as are leads from a dermatologist. The ISHRS and the websites listed above are also good starting places.

Hair-System Specialists

If you are interested in a cosmetic hair addition, a personal reference is, of course, the best place to begin. Do you know anyone who wears an addition that you find natural looking and to your liking? If you feel comfortable enough with the person, ask where he got it. Also ask about his impression of the company, as well as the person who helped in the selection. If you have no personal contacts and must start from square one, check the Yellow Pages under "Hair Restoration" or "Hair Replacement" for centers and offices that are located in your area. As it is for locating surgeons, the Internet is another great source for listings of local retailers.

Just keep in mind that any contacts you obtain, whether from a website or a person who has had first-hand experience, are only "leads." You must check them out further, asking questions, discovering what the providers can offer, and getting a sense of their honesty and professionalism.

EVALUATING A PROVIDER

Once you have obtained the names of transplantation surgeons or hair-system providers, it's on to the next step—evaluation. Just one

word of advice before you begin. During your meetings and consultations, always try to be aware of the hype and misinformation
that, unfortunately, is prevalent in the hair-replacement industry.
In this chapter, we will point out some of the most common ways
in which you can be misled.

The Consultation

The consultation is a time for learning more about the provider's
hair-replacement procedures or the products that he or she represents. It is also a time to learn of the provider's beliefs, goals, and
commitment to ethical business practices.

Before any consultation, it's important for you to know your
rights. Due to the overwhelming crush of misinformation, misleading advertising tactics, and economic pressures on physicians
and hair-addition specialists alike, your rights as a consumer have
been somewhat compromised. You do, however, have the right to
have your questions answered, the provider's plan explained to
you in writing, feel no pressure about the decision you're making,
and much more. The inset on page 164 offers a detailed list of your
rights as a hair-replacement client.

To further ensure that your rights are protected, be prepared
for your consultations. Prior to each meeting, compile a list of
questions that you would like addressed. Reviewing the information in this book will help you formulate some of your queries.
Always ask the provider if the replacement method you are interested in will work with your particular type of hair loss; if you're
unsure of your type, first see a doctor who specializes in hair loss
for a proper diagnosis.

Arrange to bring a friend or family member with you during
the meeting. This second pair of ears will help you remember information and verify what the provider has said. Furthermore, being
detached from the situation, he or she is likely to be objective in
helping you evaluate that information. If you are unable to bring
someone with you (or prefer not to), it might be a good idea to bring
a tape recorder. Be sure the provider knows that you will be record-
ing the conversation. He or she shouldn't have any objections.

Finally, try to avoid "shopping" for a hair replacement when
you are feeling particularly upset or emotional over your hair loss.

The Hair-Replacement Client's Bill of Rights

Over the years, we have discovered that many of our patients had been grossly misinformed and even mistreated by surgeons and people posing as experts in the field of hair replacement. It became obvious that many consumers simply didn't know what to expect or how to determine if a provider was forthright and ethical. One of our primary objectives when writing this book was to clearly explain your rights as a consumer, and to heighten your awareness of what to expect from a hair provider. To this end, we created the following Bill of Rights. Some of these rights apply to surgical hair replacement, others to nonsurgical options, and some to both.

As a prospective client, you have a right to:

■ A provider who is experienced and knowledgeable; someone who makes you feel comfortable and at ease.

■ As many consultations as necessary until all of your questions are answered.

■ Bring your spouse, friend, sibling, or anyone else to the consultations.

■ A thorough explanation of the provider's plan, whether a hair addition or surgery, before making a commitment. Especially in the case of surgery, you should expect a clear understanding of the procedure—of each step involved. Will there be transplants? If so, what kind of grafting is planned? How many sessions will be needed to achieve the desired results?

■ Meet and talk with your surgeon prior to the day of the surgery, not only on the day of the procedure itself.

■ Be informed of the possible complications of the surgical procedure, or drawbacks of the hair addition you are considering.

■ Full disclosure of the surgeon or provider's training and experience.

■ Meet and talk with some of the provider's other clients or patients.

■ Read the consent form at your leisure without feeling rushed, and understand it before signing.

■ Make your decision without feeling pressured by sales tactics.

It may prompt you to make a hasty decision—one that you may regret later on. If you are considering a surgical procedure, keep in mind that, unlike other forms of surgery, there is never a medical advantage to perform hair-restoration procedures sooner rather than later. This means there's no reason to be hasty with such a major decision—remind yourself that you have plenty of time. A good decision today will be a good decision tomorrow.

Your first meeting with a physician or hair-addition provider should not be rushed—on average, it should take at least thirty minutes. During this time, you should be given a complete explanation of the surgical procedure or plan for a cosmetic hair addition in clear, nontechnical, easy-to-understand language. Using this book as a reference, you can crosscheck the information that you are given. If necessary, anything you are told verbally should be further clarified with written material and/or diagrams.

In addition to presenting all of the benefits of a procedure, a good surgeon will also discuss any potential risks and dangers, even if they are unlikely. Chapter 6 includes a thorough discussion of the potential problems associated with each surgical option. If you are opting for surgery, *never* have the procedure done on the same day as the consultation. Furthermore, *never* trust a doctor who suggests that you should! It doesn't matter if you have already consulted with a number of doctors and extensively researched the treatment; a consultation is still an information-only process. Be suspicious of any doctor who pressures you or even suggests that you sign up for surgery on the same day as the consultation. Run (don't walk) out the door.

If, however, you are seeing a doctor to get a prescription for Propecia, it is reasonable to begin the treatment the same day as the consultation. As long as the doctor has told you of the medication's potential side effects and has made you aware of when you can begin experiencing results, starting Propecia immediately is fine. During the consultation, many doctors will also offer printed materials regarding the up-to-date usage and safety precautions regarding this medication.

It is acceptable, although not recommended, to consult with a hair-addition specialist and start the fitting process on the same day. This can be done as long as you feel that all of the information has been covered, your questions have been answered satisfactorily, and you are fully aware of the terms and conditions of the contract. Most people, however, need more time to think things over. Many also prefer speaking to a number of specialists, not just one. Our point here is that you should never feel embarrassed by taking as much time as you need to make a confident decision.

After the consultation, go home and calmly assess the information. Have all your questions been answered so far? Do those answers lead you to other questions that still need to be addressed? In addition to all of the information, there's another aspect of the consultation that should be assessed—the personality of the provider. If you are like most people, you will want this person to be compassionate and caring, ethical, and willing to answer your questions, no matter how trivial. You don't want to be dealing with someone who seems hurried, on the defensive, or a fast talker. After the initial consultation, you'll probably come away with a feeling about the person. To further help in your assessment, ask yourself the following questions. Does the provider:

- Seem to understand my situation and care about my feelings?

- Show a willingness to acknowledge if he is unsure of something I have asked?

- Make me feel rushed?

- Appear willing to simply talk to and listen to me?

- Offer photos of other clients and provide an opportunity for me to meet with them?

- Explain technical procedures in a way that I can understand?

In addition to compassion and caring, professional integrity is another quality that you should expect from a surgeon or hair-addition provider. They must be willing to stand behind their work and do whatever is necessary (if possible) to satisfy you as the client. Such integrity comes from experience and a commitment to service.

Don't be surprised if more questions pop up after a consultation. Either set up another appointment with the provider to have these questions answered, or discuss them during a phone consultation. Continue this process until all of your questions have been answered satisfactorily. Remember, the consultation process is not over until *you* are ready.

Assessing the Provider's Skills

Assessing the provider's technical skills, whether this involves planting grafts or fitting clients for hair additions, is another important aspect of the evaluation. Cosmetic additions must match your natural hair in terms of color and texture. They must also be properly designed for your particular shaped head and face. Of course, transplant surgeons will be using your own hair, but even so, the proper aesthetic placement of grafts is critical for a positive result.

There are a few ways to help you evaluate a provider—by verifying his or her training and certification, reviewing photographs of past work, and meeting other clients in person to review the results with your own eyes. Of these, the most helpful approach is meeting with past clients. The other strategies, although helpful, are not sufficient to accurately judge a provider's work. Furthermore, as you will see in the discussion that follows, certification and photos of past clients may not be as helpful as you might think.

If you are considering a hair transplant and have met with past clients, but wish to further gauge a doctor's skills, you can request a test session during which the surgeon transplants a few grafts. Be aware, however, that only a small number of surgeons offer this option.

Training and Certification

When choosing a doctor to perform hair-replacement surgery, the surgeon's credentials are one means of determining his ability. Just keep in mind that credentials may mean less than you think.

To date, there is no board certification credited by the American Board of Medical Specialties in the field of hair-restoration surgery, nor is there any accreditation in any other country in the world. We know of board-certified doctors with surgical training in specialized areas—cardiology, dermatology, facial plastic surgery, otolaryngology (ENT), and general plastic surgery—who also practice surgical hair rearrangement.

The American Board of Hair Restoration Surgery (ABHRS) is a recently formed board for doctors specializing in surgical hair restoration. To be accepted, the surgeon must have completed a certain number of procedures over a three-year period; he or she must also pass both a written and an oral examination. This board, however, is not recognized by the American Board of Medical Specialties and, like any board, does not certify more than a basic level of knowledge. Board certification by the ABHRS means that a doctor has met the minimum requirements of technical knowledge and understanding in the field as shown by an examination. However, unlike other specialty fields, there are no formal residency programs in hair restoration. Training may be included only as part of the curriculum of a more traditional residency training program, such as dermatology. While we agree with the concept of board certification, it does not ensure ethical practice or superior technical skills.

Any capable doctor can learn the surgical technique of hair transplantation, but not all can understand or will take the time to learn the theoretical basis of the various treatment modalities and apply them correctly. Just as important, not every doctor has the ability to maintain an ethical, caring approach to the process of surgical hair rearrangement. Some of the worst cases we've ever seen were performed by doctors who were board certified in plastic surgery, but who did not understand the application of the technique or the aesthetic requirements of hair rearrangement—qualities that come only from hands-on experience and compassion for the patient.

Most surgeons first learn only basic techniques through exposure in residency training or an introductory course. Over time, they can learn updated or advanced techniques through *preceptorship training.* Through a preceptor—an experienced doctor who serves as both teacher and mentor—the student surgeon learns the philosophy of a doctor's practice, as well as the actual surgical techniques and the reasoning behind their use. Because preceptorship training is extremely individualized, many of these "students" choose to study with more than one surgeon to ensure that they receive a balanced approach. Attendance at conferences and other group meetings is also an invaluable part of this training because it introduces the latest technical information, and gives less-experienced doctors a chance to ask questions to a wide variety of practicing doctors.

Because hair replacement is such a rapidly changing field, a doctor's initial technical training means less and less over time. A doctor can go from being a world-leading pioneer to a student very quickly. For instance, improved procedures from 1996 to 2000 have been so great that any doctor who has not adapted them is practicing outdated techniques.

A provider's training is only as good as his or her willingness to continue to learn. To correctly evaluate this, you must ask pointed and direct questions regarding interests, dedication, and the amount of time spent in the field. The following questions (along with what we consider to be "good" or "adequate" responses in parentheses) should yield some helpful insight:

- *How many procedures have you performed?*
  A minimum of 100 is best.

- *How long have you been in practice?*
  A minimum of two to three years is good.

- *How long did you train with other doctors before you began performing the procedures?*
  One year would be ideal.

- *Why did you begin doing hair transplants?*
  Although there is no right or wrong answer to this question, the response should offer some insight into the doctor's motivation and personality.

- *Which conferences and symposiums do you attend to stay current in the field?*
  At least one of the following meetings should be attended each year: The International Society of Hair Restoration Surgery, the European Society of Hair Restoration Surgery, the DHI Live Surgery Workshop, or the World Hair Society Live Workshop.

- *How do you regard alopecia reductions?*
  Alopecia reductions should not be considered primary treatments for male pattern hair loss. They can, however, be useful procedures for repair and reconstruction.

- *What is your primary surgical orientation: follicular unit transplantation or mini/micrografting?*
  This answer will indicate the surgeon's primary method of hair transplantation. Be sure to ask how many procedures of this type he or she has performed.

- *Will you arrange for me to meet with some of your former patients who have experienced hair loss that was similar to mine, and who have completed the restoration process?*
  This answer better be "YES."

While these questions have their limitations, they are valuable because they will further help you to assess the personality and skill of the surgeon. Is he defensive, belligerent, and argumentative, or is he direct, open, and forthright when answering your questions?

Unfortunately, not all hair-transplant doctors learn their skills through preceptorship training. Some attend weekend seminars in which transplantation techniques are taught. These seminars, which are typically set up by marketing consultants, attract surgeons with advertising slogans like, "Worried about managed care? Learn an exciting direct-pay alternative." They lure doctors from other fields with the promise of high-income potential, but fail to mention the amount of experience and training that, in reality, is required to achieve a minimum level of expertise.

Just keep in mind that experience is a major key to developing good transplantation techniques. Whether the surgeon has learned the basics from a two-day seminar or from spending many months in extensive preceptorship training, he or she still needs the experience in performing the actual surgery.

Photographs of Other Patients and Clients

In the past, photographs were of great importance in the cosmetic surgery and hair-addition fields because they were the primary means by which providers could show the quality of their work. The before and after photos made up their portfolios, representing their abilities, as well as the health and vitality of their practices. Today, however, photos are not as significant as they once were. If you are considering surgery, it's important to be aware of the "complete picture" when looking at photographs—there are a number of ways in which they can be misleading. If you are an educated consumer, you won't be tricked.

With increased competition, unethical business practices are invading the field. Doctors have been known to show prospective clients photos of the patients of more experienced surgeons. Although they may not actually claim the photos are of their work, they won't say that they aren't either, causing clients to make the wrong assumption. If discovered, the providers may claim that they were simply showing the prospective patient an example of the "state-of-the-art" procedure, and did not intend for them to think the photos were of their own work.

In 1990, Dr. Marritt wrote an article entitled, "A Consumer's Guide to Choosing a Surgeon," which appeared in the American Hair Loss Council's *Hair Loss Journal*. Almost 80 percent of that article focused on evaluating hair-transplant surgeries through photographs. A surgical clinic in Berlin, Germany, took some of the photos from this article and presented them in a brochure as its own. A doctor who happened to see the brochure remembered the photos from the original journal publication, and confronted the clinic about them. The clinic decided to stop using the photos in this "less than honest" way. However, even if it had refused to stop using the unauthorized photos, there would have been no legal way of preventing their unethical practice.

National hair-replacement chains typically employ a large number of surgeons. One unethical habit that is common to some of these clinics is showing prospective clients photographs of the work of only one or two of the clinic's most skilled surgeons. You may visit a clinic's branch office in New Orleans, but might be shown photos of patients who were operated on by the company's founder, who works out of the Los Angeles office. Just because the founder's patients have gotten great results is, of course, no indication that the results you get will be equally as good. These clinics rely on the fact that this won't occur to you. Insist on seeing pictures of the work performed by the surgeon who will be operating on you.

It is also important to be aware that providers can alter the appearance of patient/client photographs. For instance, using spray-on hair or augmenting transplants with a client's thinning hair can enhance the appearance in a photo. Sometimes, photographs are taken of people with no hair loss, but who claim they were once patients or clients. In addition, computer technology allows for the digital manipulation of photographs to enhance density, soften hairlines, and remove unsightly scars. Unfortunately, it is almost impossible to tell if a photograph has been doctored in this way. One final consideration is that photographs are two-dimensional representations of a three-dimensional space, and, therefore, tend to make hair look thicker than it actually is.

Despite these deceptive practices, photographs are still useful to a limited extent. They can help verify a provider's abilities—but only when used in conjunction with seeing former clients in person. And keep in mind that legitimate close-up shots should never appear individually, but always as part of a progressive series to demonstrate that they are of the same person. Valid photographs also maintain similar lighting, angle, lens, and color throughout the series.

Beyond the technical aspects of photographs, another consideration is equally, if not more important. Specifically, does the person in the photos display any characteristics that are similar to yours? Optimally, if you are considering surgery, you should look at photos of patients with similar hair-loss patterns to yours, but whose hair and skin characteristics are even less forgiving. This person should have hair color that is the same or darker than yours, skin color that is the same or lighter than yours, hair curl that is the same or straighter than yours, hair texture that is the same or finer than yours, and complete baldness within a pattern that was the same or more extensive than yours at the onset of the transplantation process. This means that even if your hair is just thinning at this point, you should view photos of someone who had areas that were completely bald before surgery. Why? Since you will be losing more hair over time, you should see what the surgeon has done in the past with a "blank" canvas. In addition, thinning hair can hide a multitude of sins, so photos of individuals who initially had completely bald spots are helpful.

Unlike men, most women do not bald completely in any given area, so photographs of female patients are more difficult to assess. There simply aren't many completely bald female patients. So actually meeting with those who have had hair transplants becomes very important for women who are considering grafts.

If you are considering a cosmetic hair addition, photo requirements are not as strict. Although it is helpful to see a person whose hair loss represents a more difficult situation than your own, other factors are more important to assess. When looking at the client, you should be more interested in seeing if the hair addition looks natural. Is it properly shaped? How does it lay on the forehead? Finally, how does the color of the addition blend with the person's natural hair color?

If you are interested in a pharmaceutical treatment, photos really mean nothing. The product will either work for you or it won't, and no one can predict how much hair regrowth you will experience. In addition, when using medications in the way that they are indicated, you should expect no better results than those published by the drug's manufacturer. Be wary of any doctor who claims (or shows photos) that results from "his formula" are better than those of a readily available medication that can be prescribed by any physician.

Meeting Other Patients and Clients

As mentioned earlier, although viewing photos can give you an indication of a surgeon's work or the artistry of a cosmetic hair addition, it is also vital that you meet with clients in person. This is important, not only to see the actual hair replacement, but also to hear of their experiences and get a sense of how they feel about the provider's services.

If a provider refuses your request to set up a meeting with a former client, this means one of two things. Either his clients are unhappy with their results, or he doesn't want to spend the time and energy making the arrangements. Those who do poor work know that if prospective clients see it, they won't get any new patients. They may attempt to mislead you by boasting that they are so good, they work only on celebrities and important people who demand their privacy. If you are faced with such a provider, we recommend that you ask, "Do you mean that the very first patient or client you worked on after you completed your training was a movie star? Wasn't there ever a time when you had average patients before you became so famous? Can I meet with one or two of your "nonfamous" clients?" Questions like these cut through such intimidation tactics, which are aimed at denying you your rights.

Also, when arranging to meet with a former client, be sure to let the provider make the connection. Never ask for the person's contact information directly. The provider should be the one to make the introduction and arrange the meeting. We also recommend that clients talk to each other privately, not in the presence of the provider. People are more likely to be honest when they're alone.

During this meeting, in addition to focusing on the person's feelings about the provider, also ask about the procedure and his personal assessment of the results. For example, it might be helpful to ask questions such as: Did the provider follow through on his word? How did he behave during and after the process was completed? Did he maintain courteous and polite service? How is the staff? Were there any surprises during or after the procedure? Are you happy with the results? Are they what you expected? How many of the doctor's patients did you meet prior to having your surgery? What did you learn from other patients you met?

Another word of advice: you have to be cautious even when meeting former patients. Some unethical physicians have been known to transplant a small number of hairs in front of a non-bald hairline, and then claim that the patient has been "transplanted." A prospective client will see someone with a full head of hair and be impressed with what he believes came from transplantation. Because the surgeon transplanted *some* hair, legally, he can claim that the patient has been transplanted—and won't expect you to assume such a scam. So be aware of this possibility, and ask to see a photo of the person "before" the transplantation.

Always keep in mind that hair replacement—whether done through surgery or a cosmetic hair addition—is a service industry. Your needs as a client must be addressed. Any provider who is unwilling to accommodate your rational expectations is not servicing your needs appropriately. Also remember that doctors or providers, even those who are ethical, will show you only their *best* patients.

SEEING THROUGH THE HYPE

You just learned how before and after photos can be tricky and misleading. Now let's take a look at some other common gimmicks and deceptive claims that providers have used to generate business. We want you to be aware of them. They should ring a warning bell and put you on your guard.

Immediate Openings

Some doctors and clinics will try to lure clients with promises of immediate openings to begin the procedure. But ask yourself, if the provider is so fantastic, why are there openings in the surgical schedule that can accommodate you any time you want? It's quite likely that the clinic isn't bringing in enough patients to cover expenses, which puts significant pressure on the doctors or hair-addition specialists. A provider with a full schedule is in a better position to act responsibly because he is under less pressure to fill surgery time or sell more hair additions.

Start Today!

Some doctors and clinics offer special prices for anyone who is willing to start the hair-replacement process immediately. The doctor may say, "We're offering a special discount for anyone who agrees to have surgery at some point during this month," or "We'll give you an extra 100 grafts free." At this point, the question that should leap in your mind is, "Why such an offer? Doesn't he have enough business?" The field of cosmetic surgery is no place for such incentives. Even if you are buying a hair addition, you are still making a major purchase that needs to be handled seriously and calmly—not something to be rushed into.

Phone Solicitations

Phone solicitation is another promotional tool that some doctors have adopted to gain patients, once again bucking traditional medical standards. Can you imagine a doctor calling to ask if you want him to remove the bunion he noticed on your last visit? Hair-replacement clinics or private-practice surgeons may make such calls because they know that those with hair loss are often desperate and won't object to this type of inappropriate solicitation.

Completely Affordable

Would you rather have a diamond or a cubic zirconium? A Yugo or a Mercedes? Remember that you get what you pay for. Businesses typically make money in one of two ways—either by selling a huge amount of a product for a small amount of money, or by selling a small amount of a product for a large amount of money. While you may be willing to settle for a cheaper car or a piece of costume jewelry, are you willing to settle for the economical version of a hair addition or a surgical procedure?

Full Density in One Megasession. Guaranteed!

Men have all sorts of reasons for wanting surgery performed quickly. "I'm in a wedding in two months." "I'm flying to Europe for an important business deal." "Summer is coming and I want to look good at the beach." To appeal to those people who want it all—and immediately—many surgical clinics offer "super fantastic megasessions." The truth is, it just isn't possible to get complete density *and* coverage in a single session, even with follicular unit transplants. Be extremely wary of the surgeon who makes such a promise.

Unlike surgery, cosmetic hair additions do provide immediate coverage and density. However, be careful of the less than ethical provider who offers to get you an addition quickly, without the proper consultation and fitting process. You will never get a good-quality, natural-looking addition this way.

The Doctor as Artistic Genius

Good surgeons take a strictly limited set of rules and procedures coupled with sound surgical protocols and apply them when constructing hairlines or creating whorls at the crown. They are not being "artistic." They are simply copying the natural patterns found on the head. If they are anything, good surgeons are *artisans*.

Be wary of any provider, but especially of the surgeon, who claims that he is artistic. You do not want art. You want the careful and studied re-creation of what nature produced. Nature itself—not the doctor's interpretation of it—defines what is most "natural."

Testimonials

Providers of both hair-transplant surgery and hair additions sometimes use brochures and videos to present patient testimonials. Often, a former client is shown smiling proudly as he stands next to a gorgeous female. He talks about how much more confident and effective he has become at work and in his social life since he regained a full head of hair. Such talk is a powerful motivator for many prospective patients, who feel that it confirms their own expectations. The video testimonial can create a real sense of identification with only a few pictures and a few seconds of dialogue. Just remember that the people in the video may be actors whose words have been scripted and who are simply doing a job. They may have never even experienced balding. Beware!

You Can Have It All!

Don't believe any provider who implies that you won't have to make any compromises or concessions. Many men with hair loss cannot get complete coverage through surgery alone, because they do not have enough donor hair. Hair additions *can* provide full coverage, but they still may not be able to provide it "all" when it comes to undetectability or the ability to participate in certain sports. And finally, the use of pharmaceuticals cannot result in complete coverage. With hair replacement, there is always compromise.

THE CONSENT FORM

Both hair-addition companies and surgeons use a consent form as part of their standard operating procedure. It is vital that you sign this form, which ensures that you are fully informed and aware of any potential complications of the procedure. It also outlines in writing what will be happening during the process, whether it is having surgical hair rearrangement or getting a hair addition.

For hair additions, this form is actually a binding contract that lists costs, warranty information, maintenance schedules, and other important data. For surgery, it should reiterate everything that was communicated to you by the surgeon and his staff. This should include, but not be limited to, risks of the procedure, goals of the surgery, and nonsurgical options. There should be no surprises on the consent form.

If you don't agree with any of the terms on the form, discuss them with your provider and make any necessary amendments. Many points may be negotiable. For example, if the form stipulates that the provider is able to use your photos in publications, but you aren't comfortable with this, you can have this provision removed.

When having surgery, be sure to see the consent form prior to the day of the procedure. You should have enough time to go over the form carefully, noting any changes that you feel are appropriate, and having any of your questions or concerns explained or clarified. The consent form should not present any substantive information that you have not already discussed with your provider. Take the contract home and read it at your leisure to fully understand what you are (and are not) getting. These contracts can resemble car warranties, and should be double-checked for complete understanding.

Finally, always keep in mind that signing a consent form does not remove your right to hold the surgeon responsible for any problems or complications that may result from the procedure. If a surgeon does not adequately attempt to make the appropriate corrections, you'll still have legal recourse. But also remember that discretion is the better part of valor. Allow your surgeon to take care of any problems first. If you are comfortable with your surgeon and feel that he cares about you and your results, you should feel confident that he will also try to remedy any problems.

CONCLUSION

The next phase of your journey is close at hand. We recommend that you review this book carefully before your consultations. Use it as your personal reference guide. Although it may take time to find a provider who you feel has both the skills and the honesty that you are seeking, your determination and patience will be rewarded when you reach your goal of getting natural-looking, undetectable hair.

Conclusion

In an industry that continues to experience tremendous techno-logical and scientific growth, no one knows what cutting-edge pro-cedure or revolutionary new product may one day be available for the treatment of hair loss. Current scientific research is underway in the area of gene therapy and tissue engineering, more com-monly known as *cloning*. One day, there may actually be a cure for hair loss. But until that day, don't underestimate the treatment options at hand. Cosmetic hair additions, with their advanced materials and state-of-the-art construction methods, now have a more natural look and feel than ever before. Cutting-edge surgical procedures, particularly the follicular unit transplantation tech-nique, can give a person completely natural and undetectable re-sults. And although minoxidil and finasteride are currently the only FDA-approved pharmaceuticals for treating hair loss, scien-tists continue the search for breakthrough products.

It is our sincere hope that the information contained within this book has given you confidence and security in your knowledge of the many facets of hair loss—from an understanding of its phys-ical causes to a familiarity with legitimate treatment alternatives. With clarity and objectivity, you can assess each of the available treatment methods with your own specific goals and expectations in mind. Your awareness of the realities of the treatments—their capabilities as well as their limitations—will aid you tremendous-ly in making the best choice for your particular situation. During your search, always keep the following points in mind:

- You have options, including doing nothing.

- You have time. Don't rush into any decisions.

- You have knowledge regarding your condition; you will not be swayed by misinformation.

- You have complete control over the treatment you select and who will help you with that treatment.

- Because of your knowledge and control, you are empowered to make a decision based on your rational objectives.

You now have the tools to take the next step—finding the right person or treatment to help you achieve your goal. As the saying goes, give a man a fish and you have fed him for a day; teach a man to fish, and you have fed him for the rest of his life. We wish you the best of luck.

Glossary

Alopecia. General term for hair loss, of which there are many types and causes.

Alopecia areata. An autoimmune condition in which complete baldness occurs in random but clearly defined patches on the scalp.

Alopecia reduction (AR). A surgical procedure in which a bald section of the scalp is removed and then sutured closed to reduce the size of the bald area. Commonly referred to as a *scalp reduction.*

Alopecia totalis. An autoimmune condition in which complete baldness occurs over the entire scalp.

Alopecia universalis. An autoimmune condition in which complete baldness occurs over the entire body.

Anagen effluvium. Significant loss of hair during the anagen (growth) phase.

Anagen phase. The growth phase of the hair cycle, during which the follicle is actively producing a hair. At any given time, approximately 85 percent of the hairs on an individual's head are in the anagen phase, which may last from two to six years.

Androgen. General term for any male hormone. Testosterone is the primary androgen.

Androgenetic alopecia. The genetic predisposition to lose hair. In men, this is referred to as *male pattern baldness;* in women, it is called *female pattern baldness.*

Antiandrogens. Agents that block the function of male hormones; some antiandrogens are effective in treating hair loss.

181

AR. *See* Alopecia reduction.

Arteriovenous fistula. A small blood-filled sac that forms when a vein heals to a nearby artery. It feels like a small balloon beneath the skin.

Base. The main structural component of a hair addition, giving it shape and contour. The "hair" of an addition is attached to the base.

Beading. An attachment method for cosmetic hair additions in which existing hair is pulled through eyelets at the edge of the base and then secured with small metal beads.

Bulb. The bulb-shaped lower portion of the hair follicle, containing cells that determine the width of the fully grown hair.

Catagen phase. The transitional phase of the hair cycle that follows the anagen (growth) phase. During this phase, which lasts from one to six weeks, the follicle ceases to produce hair.

Circumferential scar. Located along the top border of the fringe area; this type of scar is the result of an extensive scalp lift.

Cobblestoning. The lumpy appearance of the scalp, resulting from standard grafts or minigrafts that don't heal evenly with the scalp's surface.

Compression. *See* Graft compression.

Crown. The top or highest part of the head. Also called the *vertex.*

Cyberhair. A revolutionary synthetic nylon fiber that looks and feels like real hair.

Density. Term referring to the visual thickness of hair or the number of hairs in a given area of the scalp.

Dermal papilla. A specialized group of cells located at the base of a follicle that are believed to regulate hair growth.

DHT. *See* Dihydrotestosterone.

Diffuse patterned alopecia. A condition in which the hair thins noticeably, but not to complete baldness. The thinning occurs in the same characteristic pattern as male pattern baldness.

Diffuse unpatterned alopecia. A condition that is characterized by general thinning of the hair over the entire head (including the fringe area). The hair loss usually occurs equally throughout the scalp, but in rare instances, it happens in random patches. This condition is much more common in women than in men.

Dihydrotestosterone (DHT). The male hormone responsible for male pattern baldness, acne, and prostate enlargement. DHT also stimulates hair growth on the face and body.

Donor dominance. The principle that transplanted hair will maintain the characteristics of the area from which it comes (the hair-bearing donor area), rather than the area into which it is transplanted (the bald recipient area). This principle accounts for the fact that transplanted hair will continue to grow after it is placed in a bald area.

Donor site. The hair-bearing area of the scalp. Located on the sides and/or back of the head, this area is the source of grafts for transplantation procedures.

Double-blind study. A scientific study in which neither the subjects nor the researchers know which subjects are taking the drug and which are taking the placebo. This type of study is conducted to ensure objective results.

Dutasteride. A DHT blocker (developed by GlaxoSmithKline) that is used in the treatment of benign prostatic hyperplasia (BPH) or enlarged prostate. Because dutasteride inhibits the formation of both types of DHT, its use may result in more hair growth (or less hair loss) than that seen with finasteride.

Female pattern baldness. *See* Androgenetic alopecia.

Finasteride. The active ingredient in the oral drug Propecia (manufactured by Merck) for the treatment of hair loss. By inhibiting the Type II 5 alpha-reductase ($5\alpha R$) enzyme, finasteride blocks the formation of Type II DHT, allowing intermediate hair follicles to enlarge and regrow terminal hairs in some individuals.

5 alpha-reductase ($5\alpha R$). The enzyme responsible for converting testosterone to dihydrotestosterone (DHT).

Flap surgery. *See* Skin flap surgery.

Follicle. A small pouch-like structure below the surface of the skin in which a hair is produced.

Follicular unit. A naturally occurring group of hair follicles. Typically, each unit contains 1 to 4 hairs.

Follicular unit transplantation (FUT). A hair-transplant method in which intact follicular units are grafted into balding areas.

Forelock. The hair located on the front third of the scalp—on or above the forehead.

Fringe. The hair remaining on the sides and back of the head after extensive hair loss.

Full-head bonding. Technique in which the entire base of a cosmetic hair addition is attached to the scalp with an adhesive that lasts longer than the type used in removable additions. Also called a *nonsurgical graft.*

FUT. *See* Follicular unit transplantation.

Graft Compression. A complication that can result when large grafts containing many follicular units are placed into a site, and the connective tissue compresses the grafts, causing the follicles to lie close to one another. The resulting appearance resembles a "bundle" or "rope" of hair emerging from a single graft site.

Grafting. *See* Hair transplantation.

Grafts. Hairs that are removed from the donor area of the scalp and transplanted into a balding area. Graft types include standard grafts, minigrafts, micrografts, and follicular units.

Hair additions. General term used to describe hair extensions, weaves, integrations, fusions, and nonsurgical grafts. Also called *hair systems.*

Hair shaft. The part of a hair that projects from the surface of the skin or scalp; it's the part of the hair you can see.

Hair systems. *See* Hair additions.

Hair transplantation. The method of moving hair from the permanent donor area of the scalp to a balding area.

Halo formation. A possible consequence that occurs after hair is transplanted into a bald area, but hair loss continues in the surrounding area. The eventual result is a "halo" of bald skin that forms around the grafted area.

Integration. *See* Weaving.

Intermediate hairs. Hairs that are somewhat thinner, softer, shorter, and lighter in color than terminal hairs, but not quite vellus-like.

Keloids. Large raised scar formations.

Ketoconazole. An antifungal ingredient with antiandrogenetic properties found in Nizoral, a dandruff shampoo.

Loniten. A blood pressure medication (developed by Upjohn) whose active ingredient is minoxidil.

Loose scalp. A scalp characterized by skin that moves easily.

Ludwig Scale. Commonly used scale for the classification of female pattern baldness.

Male pattern baldness. *See* Androgenetic alopecia.

Micro Point Linking. A process in which synthetic Cyberhair is linked to existing hair without adhesives, weaves, clips, or surgery.

Micrograft. A very small graft that is no larger than 1 millimeter and contains 1 or 2 hairs.

Minigraft. A small graft, usually square in shape, that ranges from 1 to 2 millimeters in size, and contains 3 to 12 hairs.

Minoxidil. The first FDA-approved drug for the treatment of hair loss. Initially manufactured by Upjohn as Rogaine, minoxidil is a topical medication that slows hair loss and/or stimulates hair growth in some individuals.

Monk's spot. Term for a bald spot on the crown area of the head.

Nonsurgical graft. *See* Full-head bonding.

Norwood Scale. Commonly used scale for the hair-loss classification of male pattern baldness.

Perimeter bonding. A technique in which the base of a cosmetic hair addition is bound to existing fringe hair with an adhesive.

Plugginess. The resulting appearance of a hair transplant in which the grafts aggregate in small areas (often in unnatural-looking rows), instead of being placed in a more diffuse natural growth pattern.

Poaching. The process of obtaining viable follicular units from a seemingly used-up donor area.

Propecia. The brand name of an FDA-approved oral medication (manufactured by Merck), containing 1 milligram of finasteride, for the treatment of hair loss.

Proscar. The brand name of a medication (manufactured by Merck), containing 5 milligrams of finasteride, for the treatment of benign prostatic hyperplasia (BPH) or enlarged prostate.

Prostate-specific antigen (PSA). A marker in the blood that is elevated in individuals with prostate cancer.

Pruning. The process of removing follicles from a previously transplanted graft to improve the appearance of plugginess or compression.

PSA. *See* Prostate-specific antigen.

Recipient area. The general area of the scalp in which grafts are placed.

Recipient site. The scalp location in which a single graft is placed.

Recombinant follicular unit transplantation. Transplantation technique in which multiple follicular units (such as a 1-hair and 3-hair unit, or three 1-hair units) are placed into a single recipient site. This method achieves greater density in a single session than standard FUT surgery.

Retin-A. The brand name of the generic drug tretinoin, a prescription medication used for treating acne. It is sometimes combined with minoxidil to enhance absorption into the scalp.

Rogaine. Upjohn's brand name for minoxidil, the first FDA-approved drug for the treatment of hair loss. Available without a prescription, Rogaine comes in 2% and 5% strengths.

Scalp expander. A balloon-like device that is placed under the scalp, and then expanded with saline to stretch the skin. Its use may facilitate an alopecia reduction or scar-reduction surgery.

Scalp extender. A device that is placed under a hair-bearing area of the scalp to stretch it. Once stretched, the skin is used to cover the portion of bald skin that has been removed during an alopecia reduction.

Scalp lifting. A procedure in which the hair-bearing fringe area is surgically separated from the deeper tissue layers of the skull and upper neck. During an alopecia reduction, the loose skin is then pulled towards the top of the scalp, redraped over the area from which the bald skin has been removed, and then sewn into place.

Scalp reduction. *See* Alopecia reduction.

Scar revision. A surgical procedure for decreasing the size of a scar to enhance its appearance.

Sealants. General term for adhesives that are used to attach cosmetic hair systems to the scalp.

Senile alopecia. A condition of thinning hair that occurs with age.

Shock loss. Loss of the existing hair that surrounds a new graft that may be caused by a temporary lack of blood to the area or from inflammation during the healing process. Regrowth should occur two to three months following the transplant.

Skin flap surgery. A surgical procedure in which a relatively large piece of hair-bearing skin from the side of the head is moved to a bald area. One side of this flap remains attached to the scalp to maintain the original blood supply.

Slot correction. A surgical procedure for decreasing the visibility of a slot deformation.

Slot deformation. Abnormal hair direction and visible scar along the length of the head; this "deformation" is caused by alopecia reduction surgery in which the opposing fringes are brought together at the top of the head.

Standard grafts. Relatively large grafts (approximately 4 millimeters in diameter—a little smaller than a pencil eraser) that are round in shape and contain around 16 to 20 hairs. Standard grafts were used in the first transplants, but due to improved transplantation techniques, they are rarely used today.

Stretch-back. A common phenomenon following alopecia reduction surgery in which the "stretched" hair-bearing fringe returns to its original position.

Telogen effluvium. Significant loss of hair during the telogen (resting) phase.

Telogen phase. The five- to six-week resting phase in the life cycle of a hair, during which the follicle shrinks, and the hair is "pushed out" by a new hair in the anagen phase. Hair in the telogen phase can also be shed or lost during brushing or washing.

Temporal hair. The hair that is located in the area above the temples.

Temporal recession. Hair loss in the area above the temples; this is often the first sign of male pattern baldness.

Terminal hairs. Fully developed hairs with color and texture that continue to grow after they are cut.

Three hair-bearing flaps transposition. A procedure designed to correct a slot deformation by re-establishing normal hair direction through the cutting and placement of three skin flaps.

Traction alopecia. Hair loss caused by prolonged physical tension on the hair. This can occur from wearing very tight braids, ponytails, corn rows, or certain hair additions that are attached to existing hair.

Transplants. *See* Grafts.

Triangle wedge resection. A surgical procedure, similar to a small alopecia reduction, in which unwanted hair-bearing skin over the temples is removed to create a properly shaped hairline.

Trichotillomania. A psychological condition in which a person (typically female) is compelled to pluck or pull hair from the scalp, eyebrows, or eyelashes.

Vellus hairs. Hair that is softer and finer in texture, and lighter in color than terminal hairs. They are often found at the very front of the hairline or in the area between a bald area and a hair-bearing area. Often referred to as "peach fuzz."

Vertex. The top or highest part of the head. Also called the *crown*.

Weaving. Method of attaching a hair addition by sewing it to tightly braided existing hair on the perimeter of the balding area. Also called hair *integration*.

White sidewalls. Unnaturally wide hairless areas that are located along the nape of the neck or around the ears—the possible result of scalp lifting.

Widow's peak. V-shaped point that is formed by the hair in the middle of the forehead.

Advocacy Groups

Whether you are looking for general information about hair loss, have questions about the legitimacy of a particular hair product, or need physician referrals in your area, the following professional organizations and consumer groups will be able to help. Keep in mind that any contacts you obtain, whether from one of the following groups listed below or from a person who has had first-hand experience, are only "leads." You must check them out further, asking questions, discovering what they can offer, and getting a sense if they can meet your personal needs.

Professional Organizations

The International Society of Hair Restoration Surgery (ISHRS)
13 South 2nd Street • Geneva, IL 60134
Phone: 800-444-2737 • 630-262-5399 • Fax: 630-262-1520
E-mail: info@ishrs.org • Web: www.ISHRS.org

This nonprofit voluntary organization of over 700 hair-restoration specialists provides consumers with the most current information on hair-restoration surgery. It also offers names of physicians in your area who are ISHRS members in good standing. Doctor profiles include their contact information, as well as educational and professional backgrounds, and any achievements in the field.

The American Academy of Dermatology (AAD)
PO Box 4014 • Schaumburg, IL 60168-4014
Phone: 847-330-0230 • Fax: 847-330-0050
Web: www.aad.org

This association is the largest, most representative of practicing dermatologists in the United States. Among its offerings, the AAD provides current information on conditions of the skin and hair, and names of local board-certified dermatologists.

Consumer Websites

www.TheBaldTruth.com

This site is headed by Spencer David Kobren—considered the country's "most prominent and effective hair loss consumer/patient advocate." He is the founder and director of The Bald Truth Foundation, ". . . dedicated to consumer advocacy, education and funding research regarding hair loss." This site is packed with the most current information regarding all areas of hair loss, including the latest research and treatment options. Its "scambusters" blows the whistle on the "too-good-to-be-true" products in the marketplace.

www.HairLossHelp.com

In addition to basic information on hair loss, this site includes interviews with leading industry experts, an active message board, live chats, and product ratings.

www.HairLossTalk.com

Among its many offerings, this consumer hair loss information website has a resource library, offers product reviews and consumer alerts, and sponsors online chats and message boards.

www.HairTransplant Network.com

One of the main features of this site is that it provides contact and background information of surgeons who have "demonstrated a track record of performing outstanding hair transplantation . . . chosen and recommended on the merits of their credentials and end results." It was created as an online community in which people could openly exchange information and learn about various clinics and procedures.

www.Keratin.com

This site offers information on a wide variety of hair-related subjects from common pattern baldness to rare inflammatory alopecias. It has an active message board that provides a forum for discussions of hair biology, hair loss, hirsutism, and hair products.

www.Regrowth.com

This site offers a wealth of information on hair loss and its up-to-date treatment options. It also features forums, articles, conference dates, and surveys.

Bibliography

Bernstein, R., W. Rassman, W. Szaniawski, and A. Halperin. "Follicular Transplantation." *International Journal of Aesthetic and Restorative Surgery*, Vol. 3 (1995), No. 2, pp.119–132.

Harris, J. "Hair Transplantation" in *ENT Secrets, 2nd Edition*. Jafek, B., and B. Murrow (eds). Philadelphia: Hanley & Belfus, 2001.

Inaba, M., and Y. Inaba. *Androgenetic Alopecia: Modern Concepts of Pathogenesis and Treatment*. Tokyo: Springer-Verlag, 1996.

Kaufman, K., E. Olsen, D. Whiting, et al. "Finasteride in the Treatment of Men With Androgenetic Alopecia. Finasteride Male Pattern Hair Loss Study Group." *Journal of the American Academy of Dermatology*, Vol. 39 (4 Pt. 1) (October 1998), pp. 578–589.

Marritt, E., and R. Konior. "Patient Selection, Candidacy, and Treatment Plan for Hair Replacement Surgery." *Facial Plastic Surgery Clinics of North America*, Vol. 7 (November, 1999), No. 4.

Norwood, O. "Male Patern Baldness: Classification and Incidence." *Southern Medical Journal*, Vol. 68 (November 1975), No. 11, pp.1359–1365.

Olsen, E. (ed). *Disorders of Hair Growth. Diagnosis and Treatment*, New York: McGraw-Hill, 1994.

Olsen, E. (ed). "Treatment of Androgen-Related Disorders." *Dermatologic Therapy*, Vol. 8 (1998).

Olsen, E., M. Weiner, I. Amara, and E. DeLong. "Five-year Follow-up of Men with Androgenetic Alopecia Treated with Topical Minoxidil." *Journal of the American Academy of Dermatology,* Vol. 22 (1990), pp. 643–646.

Olsen, E., M. Weiner, E. DeLong, and S. Pinnell. "Topical Minoxidil in Early Male Pattern Baldness." *Journal of the American Academy of Dermatology,* Vol. 13 (1985), pp.185–192.

Unger, W. (ed). *Hair Transplantation, 3rd Edition.* New York: Marcel Dekker, 1995.

Whiting, D., and F. Howsden. *Color Atlas of Differential Diagnosis of Hair Loss.* Cedar Grove: Canfield Publishing, 1996.

About the Authors

James A. Harris, MD, FACS, is a facial plastic surgeon in Denver, Colorado. His practice, Hair Sciences Center of Colorado, is limited exclusively to follicular unit hair transplantation. Dr. Harris graduated with honors from the University of Colorado School of Medicine in 1989 and completed his residency in Otolaryngology/Head and Neck Surgery in 1994. He currently serves as a Clinical Instructor of Hair Transplantation at the University of Colorado Health Sciences Center, Department of Otolaryngology/Head and Neck Surgery.

Before launching his private practice, Dr. Harris studied with physicians throughout the United States and completed a mini-fellowship in follicular unit hair transplantation. He was mentored by Dr. Emanuel Marritt, a recognized pioneer in the sub-specialty of mini-micrografting, and became the successor of his practice in 1999. Doctors Harris and Marritt continue to collaborate in consumer education efforts.

Dr. Harris is a Diplomate of the American Board of Otolaryngology, fellow of the American College of Surgeons, and member of the American Academy of Otolaryngology and the International Society of Hair Restoration Surgery (ISHRS). A researcher and the author of numerous medical journal publications, Dr. Harris regularly presents at the ISHRS annual conferences and frequently serves as a resource for broadcast and print media. His articles on follicular unit transplantation have been featured in many consumer publications. Dr. Harris's website is www.hsccolorado.com.

Emanuel Marritt, MD, is a dermatologic surgeon who, for over twenty-five years, limited his practice exclusively to the treatment of male pattern baldness. Before his retirement in 1999, he served as an Associate Clinical Professor in the Department of Otolaryngology/Head and Neck Surgery at the University of Colorado Health Sciences Center in Denver, Colorado. He is board certified by the American Board of Cosmetic Surgery and a fellow of both the American and International Societies of Dermatologic Surgery.

Dr. Marritt authored the first report in the United States on single hair transplantation for the *Journal for Dermatologic Surgery.* Since then, he has published over a dozen original articles on surgical hair replacement and contributed numerous chapters for contemporary surgical texts on the subject. He has been an internationally recognized authority and invited lecturer at professional symposia for more than two decades.

As the field of medical and surgical hair replacement has evolved from a small sub-specialty to a big business industry, Dr. Marritt has increased his efforts to advise and inform the public. A strong consumer advocate, he has appeared on such national television programs as *Today, Hour Magazine, CBS This Morning,* and *Dateline NBC.*

Index